MY JOURNEY THROUGH DEPRESSION

A Pastor's Story

by
Pastor David Robertson

Strategic Book Publishing and Rights Co.

Strategic Book Publishing and Rights Co.
12620 FM 1960, Suite A4-507
Houston, TX 77065
www.sbpra.com

ISBN: 978-1-60976-235-3

Design: Dedicated Book Services, Inc. (www.netdbs.com)

Dedication

This book is dedicated to my wife, Linda, who never gave up on me even in the lowest moments for both of us. You are truly heaven sent! And I am indebted to my Lord and Savior, Jesus Christ, who performed a miracle of healing in me in one moment of time! Without Him, I would not be alive today. He gets all the glory, honor, and praise!

Foreword

This story is one of the most brutally honest and most transparent that has come along in recent years. A friend of mine, Jamie Buckingham, an award-winning magazine and newspaper columnist and who was one of the most widely-read Christian writers of his day, (he was also editor-in-chief of Ministries Today magazine, editor-at-large for Charisma magazine, and author of numerous books), taught us in his speaking and writing about the value of "telling it all." This approach disarms the enemy. You leave nothing for the devil to use against you.

David and Linda Robertson have lived through the most difficult tests and trials of a marriage and have come through on the other side successfully. They may be battle worn and weary, but telling their story not only energizes them, but assures each of us that the truth will set you free! It also offers a degree of insurance that it won't happen again.

When they came to me, God had already prepared them for deliverance. It seemed immediate, but God was already at work. David had made up his mind to come home to Linda and to the call that God had on his life.

I have no doubt the future holds more ministries for them than in previous years. All of these experiences have tempered them and enabled them to reach a depth spiritually that they previously had not known.

Anybody reading this book will be able to relate to many of the same things David and Linda went through and will be helped and encouraged by it.

God Bless,
Pastor Buddy Tipton
Central Assembly of God
Vero Beach, Florida

Acknowledgments

My deepest thanks to the following:

My best friend and beautiful wife, Linda Robertson, for your invaluable encouragement and suggestions, but even more, for your love.

My spiritual father, Pastor Buddy Tipton, for your kindness and wisdom have proven what God can do through a life yielded to His complete will.

My dear friends, John and Sandy Alford, for your constant prayers and support.

My close friend, Philip McPherson, for your constant checking up on me, week after week, until the battle was won!

Introduction

Depression is defined by Webster as "a psychoneurotic or psychotic disorder marked especially by sadness, inactivity, difficulty in thinking and concentration, a significant increase or decrease in appetite and time spent sleeping, feelings of dejection and hopelessness, and sometimes suicidal tendencies."

It is my hope and prayer that through my story, others who have experienced depression will get a sense of hope and comfort from our great and loving God. It is also my desire that those of you who are caregivers to one going through depression will not give up, but instead have hope that God can heal and restore.

In the fall of 2007, I began a journey that would last until February 8, 2009. I went into a state of severe clinical depression. I had three doctors working with me at this time, and all three diagnosed me with the exact same condition. I had no idea what had hit me! All I knew was that for most of that time—nearly a year and a half—I felt extreme pain, anxiety, and hopelessness—and it was a twenty-four/seven phenomenon. It was nonstop! No one understood it at first— not me, not my wife, not my family, and especially not my church family. They all thought I was playing some sort of game or was simply going through a mid-life crisis. How wrong they were!

Part 1:

MY STORY

(Pastor Dave's Story)

Chapter 1

My depression first started to show in the form of anxiety. This was in the late fall of 2007. There were times that right in the middle of an activity or even resting I would feel all jittery, anxious, and nervous. My heart would start to race, and I felt as if something had me by the throat. I would begin to pray, and the feeling would eventually subside. It then got increasingly hard for me to be around other people. I found myself isolating myself from others and just wanting to be alone. It wasn't that I disliked anyone or was angry at them; I just wanted to be left alone. This was totally out of character for me. Being a pastor, at that time for twelve years, I was very much a people person. Like my dad, I didn't know a stranger. I could talk to anyone of any age and relate; and I honestly loved it!

At Christmas time of that year the depression had really started to kick in. I remember sitting in my easy chair with all my family in the room. My three boys were there with my grandkids sitting at my feet and playing. It was a picture perfect moment until this anxiety attack hit me so hard that I got up from my easy chair, and without a word, went to my car and drove away. I drove for awhile before ending up in the parking lot of Wal-Mart and didn't return home until 3:00 the next morning.

As the anxiety attacks became more frequent and more severe, I began to be extremely discouraged and depressed. And I didn't know why! I had everything to live for—a beautiful and loving wife; a church family I loved very much; three great boys I was proud of; four beautiful grandchildren I adored; a successful teaching career of twenty-seven years at that time; and to top it all off, the opportunity to fulfill God's will for my life up until that time—to serve Him in leading many souls to Christ!

I began to experience pain I didn't know a person could ever go through. I began to ache inside and didn't know why. It was the same sort of pain I experienced on January 13,

2003, the day they called me out of a workshop at school and informed me that my mom had been killed instantly in an automobile accident, only this pain would not go away. It built and built until I was absolutely miserable. It was now occurring every day, all day. I began to isolate myself more and more. I would go for long drives for extended periods of time and turn the music up as loud as I could stand it in order to try and drown out the feelings I was having. I began sleeping in shopping center parking lots, particularly Wal-Mart and Walgreen's. I also began to withdraw from the people I loved the most.

Chapter 2

I knew my behavior was not right. I knew that "normal" people didn't leave and sleep in parking lots and end up being gone for hours and hours alone and away from friends and family. I knew something was wrong, but really didn't know what it was. I therefore began to blame those around me. I become more withdrawn, angry, and sullen. I figured somehow the pain I felt must have been caused by everyone else. Then I did something I hadn't done in over twenty years—I began to drink. I started with a little at a time, but over the months it became more and more. I have since come to realize it is what doctors call self-medicating. People who are in depression often begin to drink or take drugs in order to blunt the pain that they are experiencing.

In February of 2008, I went to see my family physician. I explained what was going on with me, and he immediately recognized the signs and symptoms of depression. He put me on an anti-depressant, but it didn't even phase me. I believe, and my wife agrees, that it actually made me feel worse. My behavior was becoming more and more erratic; and I would go into fits of anger at the smallest thing, always perceiving someone was against me or after me.

In March of 2008, my wife, Linda, came to me and told me that she didn't know how our marriage would survive if I did not get some sort of help. In my pain I believed she wanted a divorce, that she wanted to be rid of me. I know now this wasn't true. She was simply desperate to get help for me and realized that at some point it would destroy our marriage if I didn't get help. I was falling fast. My pain continued. I tried to talk to different individuals, especially some of the men at my church, but they really didn't understand what was happening to me. They knew something was wrong, but none of them had any idea what depression was. They were as helpless as I was in the face of this "monster" that was tearing me down.

People do not really understand it until they themselves have experienced it. Like any other situation we go through, if someone has gone through it, he or she can feel your pain and know it is real. I have since found out that some of my congregation even believed I was going through a "mid-life crisis" or even worse, making it all up and playing some sort of game. I don't blame them now for not understanding. I would have had a hard time myself believing it had I not been the person experiencing it.

Linda set up a doctor's appointment for me in March of 2008 with a Christian psychiatrist. I went and for the next several months actually began to meet on a regular basis with two different ones. At first they did a complete mental health evaluation of me, and the results came back very pointed and strong. I was suffering from a mental illness—I had severe clinical depression. Not only was I diagnosed with depression, but they also found I had Attention Deficit Disorder and was bipolar!

Wow—now I was really depressed! But how and why had this happened to me? They immediately saw a plan of recovery for me, but I felt totally abandoned by God. How could God let this happen to me? I reasoned that I had been a faithful servant for years! How could God let this happen at a time when the church was growing, souls were being saved, lives were being restored? So I began to ask the age old question—why me, God? Then I began to get angry at God for what I perceived to be failure on His part to heal me and for not allowing me to have my life back. I felt He had stolen from me and then abandoned me. How wrong I was.

Chapter 3

What caused all this to begin with? First of all, I was working two full-time jobs. I had already been teaching school for fifteen years when we started the church. Not only was I teaching at that time, but I was the varsity basketball coach at the local high school. When we started the church in November of 1995, we had no idea that the tiny congregation of nine members meeting in a little community center would grow so quickly. Within four years we had purchased ten acres of land with cash and built a beautiful sanctuary/multipurpose building on it. Then we had to build again the following year in order to extend our opportunities for discipleship through Sunday School and children's ministries.

Along with all the growth came an increasing amount of responsibility for me as a pastor to meet the needs of a growing congregation. As I began to pray about what God wanted me to do, I felt Him leading me to give up my position as head coach to be able to spend more time with ministry needs. It was a heart rending decision at that time, since I was in the middle of building a program that I had started two years earlier and was committed to.

Any coach who has a heart for his players and the program he is building grows strong bonds with his players, which extend for years to come and even a lifetime. It was no different for me, thus making it an extremely difficult announcement for all of us. As time went on, we began to hire more staff positions to lighten the load and meet ministry needs. All this was wonderful and God was teaching me how to train up young leaders and release them to do ministry.

Then the second thing happened. It was just an innocent thing, but it kick started my depression. In the fall of 2007 I started taking blood pressure medicine. One of the side effects of certain blood pressure medicines is that it causes depression in approximately eighty percent of patients who start taking it. This can range from very slight to extremely severe elevations. I learned this when my physician

6

diagnosed me with my depression. Not knowing it, I had al-ready been mentally and physically exhausted from years of working two full-time jobs. Now all I needed was a catalyst to put me over the edge—and over the edge it sent me!

As if that were not enough, in January of 2008, I had a blood test done to get me ready for a colonoscopy. I have this done at least every other year since 2003 when they found and removed cancerous polyps in my colon. What they found this time scared them to the point of having me trans-ported immediately to Tampa Medical Center via ambulance in order to save my life. This episode sent me on a three month journey of even deeper mental anguish and depres-sion than I had known before.

Chapter 4

In January of 2008, I went in for my blood test. This was to be a simple procedure. I've done it many times before. I received a call a few days later saying I needed to go in again to have my blood drawn. There was something wrong with the first test because my INR number was way too high. There must be something wrong with that first test. The INR number measures how thick or thin your blood is. They said the first test was impossible, because the test showed my blood to be so thin that I shouldn't even be alive, so they needed another test. I went in and had more blood drawn.

I remember exactly where I was a few days later when I received a frantic call from the emergency room. I was standing in my classroom at the Freshman Campus where I had taught ninth graders for the last ten years. It was a teacher's work day, so no students were there that day. A call from the hospital was transferred to my room via the main office. The nurse on the other end said I needed to drop everything I was doing and come in immediately to the hospital emergency room. My blood test showed I needed immediate care. For some reason I remained calm and really didn't see the big deal. I took my time getting my room ready for the next time I was to be in school when I received another call. This time from Doctor Mavroides, my family physician, telling me I needed to come in to the emergency room immediately.

Upon hearing my physician tell me to come in, I informed the main office of the school that I was leaving to go to the hospital, but instead proceeded to go home. I went home in order to shower and shave, not knowing how long I might be at the hospital. I figured maybe a couple of hours or so, and I wanted to be clean and presentable!

After showering, I was standing in front of the sink shaving when I received another call on my cell phone. It was another nurse asking me where I was and what I was doing at that moment. I told her I would be there shortly, that I was shaving. She literally screamed over the phone in panic and told me not to shave anymore. She said if I were to cut myself even slightly, I could bleed to death on the spot! It still didn't register with me what the big deal was! I said I would be there shortly, hung up with her, and calmly finished shaving! I packed a small overnight bag and then went to the hospital.

When I walked into the emergency room, they were already waiting for me. They bypassed all the paperwork stuff and proceeded to put me in a room. (So you see, they can wait to do the paperwork if they really want to!) Then the doctor came in along with a specialist and nurses and proceeded to tell me that my blood was so thin that even the slightest bump, bruise, or cut could cause me to bleed to death. After several tests they found I lacked Factor 7, a vital clotting factor in the blood. Without it a person can literally bleed to death in a matter of minutes. They didn't understand why I was even still alive. Then I started to worry!

They made arrangements for me to be transported to Tampa General by ambulance, where they had experience treating people with blood disorders. They gave specific instructions to the paramedics to get me there as quickly as possible, but not to jostle or cause me to be bumped in any way, fearing I could bleed to death on the spot. It took three long hours to get there. In the meantime they had given me a shot of vitamin K to try to thicken my blood temporarily. I arrived in Tampa sometime after midnight and was immediately given a room in ICU.

They began taking blood from me through the IV, which had already been placed in my arm and kept me up for the next couple of hours checking on me and taking more blood samples. Around 3:00 a.m. a doctor came in and informed me that they were releasing me. He said my INR number was still high, but not high enough to keep me and do more tests. Evidently, the shot of vitamin K caused my blood to test within a high normal range for a short period of time. He then told me they needed my bed and to be out in fifteen minutes. I asked if I could stay and rest somewhere, that I had been transported by ambulance from Okeechobee and knew no one in Tampa. No family or friends were in the area. He said no. It was 3:15 a.m. and he wanted me out by 3:30 a.m. He said I could stay in the lobby like everyone else till I could get a ride home.

Wow! What a night! I was already fighting severe depression, and now I was going from dying at any moment to being kicked out of my hospital room at 3:30 in the morning, in a large city, where I knew absolutely nobody! I spent the rest of that morning in the lobby until Linda and a couple of friends were finally able to drive over to Tampa from Okeechobee and pick me up. By that time it was already 10:00 in the morning. Linda was not allowed to go to Tampa with me in the ambulance, and I had persuaded her not to drive over by herself that night, but to just wait and come with friends later the next morning. I was never so glad to see someone than when she showed up! When Doctor Mavroides found out what had taken place in Tampa, he was furious with the hospital over the way I had been treated. He proceeded to find the best blood disorder doctors available to diagnose and treat me.

This event started a several month ride of hospital visits, doctors' appointments, and ongoing blood tests to determine what was going on with me. I remember one three week period of time in which I had blood drawn at least twice a day, and sometimes three. I started feeling like a pin cushion! At one point they tried a plasma drip. What a painful experience! They had to sedate me in order to get me through it! I finally was referred to one of the most renowned blood specialists in the country. After many more tests and consultations with some of the leading blood disorder doctors in the United States, a diagnosis was finally confirmed in March of 2008. I had an extremely rare blood disorder.

Fewer than five hundred people in the United States have this same disorder. It can range from mild to severe. My case was even rarer because usually it manifests itself around the age of seven. I was missing Factor 7 from my blood; it was not a deficiency—I had no Factor 7 at all! This is the protein in the body that causes your blood to clot so as not to bleed to death when bruised or cut. Without it a person cannot live. But I was alive! How? Somehow my body had produced something in its place that the doctors cannot explain. The only question now was how stable this replacement that my body had produced was. I was informed that I would live the rest of my life with the fact that if this replacement factor ever broke down, I could be dead in a few short minutes. I could start bleeding at any moment out of the pores of my skin, my eyes, ears, nose, everywhere, because my blood would be like water. This was devastating news, particularly for an already severely depressed man! This entire trauma plunged me deeper into the black hole of depression. . . . . .

Chapter 5

March turned out to be a dreadful month! I learned not only that I was suffering from severe clinical depression, bipolar disorder, and attention deficit disorder, but also that I have a blood disorder, which could end my life at any moment! Okay, God, What's up? I asked. It now had been months since I felt the stirring of the Holy Spirit within me. I was still preaching and trying to pastor on a regular basis, but I'm definitely not feeling it! My relationship with Linda had become extremely strained due to my paranoia, anxiety, and lack of self-worth. I cried out to God for answers even as my mind was being clouded with pain and anxiety. Then I started to become angry at God thinking He had abandoned me. I had sunk so low that when I went in to see the doctor to check on my medications and have my therapy session, he almost invoked the Baker Act and had me committed. The only way I escaped this was by talking him out of it and making some concessions about my schedule.

That last week in April he told me that I had to take at least two months off from all my duties at church. If I didn't, he said, I would die. I was on the verge of a total mental breakdown and a heart attack. He told me I could keep trying to teach school, since there was only a month left and that's my major source of income; but I must take all of May and June off from church.

Do you realize how hard it was to totally walk away for that long? But I knew I must. Deep down I wanted to live, and there was a small part of me that thought that this might even help me get through this horrible episode in my life! I had three associate ministers at the time, so I put them on a rotation schedule of preaching during the time I was to be gone. I had full confidence in their abilities and knew I could trust them to do a good job and carry the load for me. I had been training and encouraging them all along, so I felt confident the church was in good hands.

During this time, the beginning of March, I began also to let my hair grow out. I had always kept it neat and trim, having it cut every other week for years. Now I was letting it grow. It was getting longer and longer. I explained it away by making all sorts of excuses to people, but down deep I knew why I was doing it. One day in June I had gone in to see my doctor. I still remember the first thing he said to me when I sat down. He looked at me and said, "Do you know why you're growing your hair long?" I told him, I did not. He said to me, "Because it's the only thing you feel like you have control of in your life. It's the one thing you can control, and no one else can tell you what to do with it. You feel like there is no other area of your life that you have any control over, especially your pain and your feelings. You feel like your life is out of control." He was right. I immediately began to cry. The tears just ran and ran. I couldn't even control them!

That's when he told me I desperately needed help. He strongly recommended to me that I admit myself to a program for two weeks in order to try to get a grip on my depression and my medication, but I refused. I knew I had to come back to the church in July and preach. For one thing, my music minister was going on vacation for five weeks, and I needed to lead the band and praise team. I could barely muster enough to even pray, let alone praise, preach, and lead a band!

July is a blur, but somehow I did it. I recycled! I preached sermons I had preached years earlier—nothing new and fresh. I went with songs all the band knew and could get through on the first practice. I was still in agonizing pain and struggling each day to just survive to the next day. I was trying different medications, but was slowly losing the battle.

All of this eventually took its toll on me. My doctor informed me again I was not going to make it if I continued. One day he sat me down and told me that before long I would begin to consider suicide if I didn't get help. I told him that there was no way! My faith wouldn't allow me. That's when he told me that he had treated many ministers just like me, and they all had said what I had said. But the time would come, he said, when my pain would be so severe that all I would be able to think of was getting relief in any way possible. He had seen some of them eventually take their own lives, having been clouded by this "monster" we call depression. But I thought somehow, if I was doing the Lord's work, He would help me. God wouldn't allow me to go that far, would He? I preached a couple more times in August, but when September came around, all the wheels began to fall off.

Chapter 6

Let me go back and clarify a few things. I don't mean to sugarcoat what has happened. If it seems sort of a manageable situation, then let me explain something—it wasn't! The summer of 2008 for Linda and me was an emotional hell! I don't know how else to say it. It began with my leaving for two weeks without her and going on a road trip that extended all the way from Daytona Beach, Florida, to the Upper Peninsula of Michigan and back. We sometimes talked but mostly would text because I couldn't handle conversation. I was so paranoid that I would sometimes scream and cry over the phone at her and then go silent for days. I put her through an emotional hell.

I remember one night I was trying to sleep in the parking lot of a little convenience store outside of Flint, Michigan, when she called. She was very concerned for my safety and wanted me to come home. I had started drinking earlier in the evening and was really messed up when she called. I would hang up on her, and then either she would call again or I would call her back. I was a mess. That went on for quite a while until I dozed off for a couple of hours. Around 1:00 in the morning I woke up and had this longing and ache to be with her. Up until this time I had been alienating myself from her and not answering my phone for days at a time. I would text her, but emotionally I was not able to hold a conversation without some sort of anger, paranoia, or anxiety spilling out. I thought that my best friend had become my enemy. That's what the devil wanted me to believe, and I bought into it for awhile!

I began to drive out of Flint around 1:00 in the morning and started south towards Florida and home. I called Linda and woke her up. I began to cry and ask her to forgive me and explained how I was feeling. She cried with me as I drove and told me how much she loved me. We talked on and off until I finally pulled over and slept in a rest area just outside of Upper Sandusky, the town in northern Ohio where I was born. When I finally woke up, I drove around my hometown for awhile and looked at the places I knew as a kid—the hospital I was born in, the park I played with my brother and cousins in. I went to the house where I first lived after I was born and then to the farm I grew up on up until I left for the Christian high school I attended in Kentucky. All the memories of my childhood came flooding back and brought me a temporary sense of calm and peace.

When I finally made it home the next day, Linda and I immediately fell into each others arms and began to try and repair the damage my disease had ravaged on us. We went to St. Augustine for a weeks vacation to get away and spend time alone sorting things out and being together. You would think that trying to work things out would bring relief, but it didn't. I was suspicious and paranoid. I took every word as critical and got angry. We had always enjoyed each other's company, but not now. Linda told me later that she prayed constantly over every word she spoke trying not to offend me. It was a mental hell for her. Satan whispered his lies and I listened. The spirits of anger and resentment clung to me. I was being ruled by anarchy in my own spirit! This spiritual attack on my soul was designed by the devil to destroy my marriage, my sanity, and ultimately, my life! The depression never left; it was trying to suck me deeper into the hole and take my wife and everything I held dear away from me forever.

The day before we were to leave we had a terrible fight. When we got back to the hotel, I left and walked for eight blocks before finding a little bar. Then I did something I hadn't done in over twenty years. I went into the bar. That was a big step for me. Remember, I am a minister of the Gospel—a servant of the King of kings. Ministers don't do this sort of thing! This was over the line for me. I had rationalized myself into buying alcohol from little out-of-the-way convenience stores where no one knew me, but to go into a bar and belly up to it was not who I was! My disease had eventually dragged me there.

I proceeded to drink as much as I possibly could. Toward the end of my drinking spree I did something that wounded

Linda deeply and hurt her for many months to come. I took off my wedding ring. I put it in my pocket and then finished that last drink. Somehow I made it back to the hotel that evening even though I had to walk back in a driving rainstorm. I didn't care about anything. I was feeling the effects of the alcohol, and for the moment it was masking my misery and pain.

I fell into bed fully clothed and rain soaked. I immediately fell asleep and didn't wake up until the next morning. Needless to say, the next day when Linda saw the ring off of my finger, she was hysterical! I had really hurt the one person in the world who loved me, wanted to help me, and knew how sick I really was. A vacation to get us back together and get me back on the road to recovery had just been yanked away in a moment's time.

Please understand something. Depression is a monster! It is a destroyer! For many people it not only can destroy your home, but it can eventually take your life if not treated or healed by God's great hand. If you have a family member who is going through this, do not hesitate to get help for them. Don't think it is just a weakness on their part and that they just need to "get a grip"! Seek medical help, but also go to God in continual prayer, interceding for them! This is a time for spiritual warfare, and that can only be fought on your knees before a holy God! Outside of the healing touch of God, it can be a long, hard process of ups and downs— with more downs than ups. I will cover this in later chapters. But make no mistake about it—those suffering from severe depression are in deep pain and distress with extreme feelings of hopelessness. They desperately need a support system from their immediate family and from their church family—they do not need judgment, criticism, and rejection!

When we arrived home, I proceeded to move some of my things out of the house and move into my mom's trailer outside of town. This started a process that would last for months—alternating times of being home and times of being away.

Chapter 7

Yes, the wheels fell off emotionally—and almost literally! In August, we had our full staff from church all back from vacation. The pressure of leading the band was off, so I chose to rotate my associate ministers in and out of the preaching schedule with me in order to relieve the pressure, especially since I was resuming teaching in mid-August.

Then it happened—the day the wheels started falling off. My depression and especially my anxiety attacks were no better. In fact, I began to have the attacks more frequently and more intensely than ever. After each episode I would sink just a little bit further into the darkness. I had a hard time sleeping. There were times I would be in front of the church preaching when all of a sudden I was gripped with an anxiety attack that would cause me to stop, take a long pause, pray quietly to myself for God's help, and then muster enough strength to continue. I came close to actually just walking out in the middle of a message on several occasions. Somehow God was still ministering through me despite my circumstances. I don't know how—but He is God!

I also had purchased a motorcycle that summer and found it extremely therapeutic to go on long rides with just myself and the open road. I hadn't ridden in almost twenty years but now found myself using it as a tool to help relieve the great pressure and stress my disease was bombarding me with. I crisscrossed the state several times just to get away to try to find relief from the torment inside. I would go to motorcycle events and try to immerse myself in the culture of riding and owning a motorcycle. I met many interesting people in the process, to say the least, but I still continued my drinking.

When I explained to my doctor what I was doing, he told me that it was a diversion tactic, which many in depression play in an attempt to escape the pain we are feeling. But when the trips were over and the car or motorcycle was parked, the "monster" was still there. It would not leave! It raised its ugly head again and again without any regard, trying to destroy me and all God had planned for me!

September ninth was a day I will never forget. After a hard day at school, I had a doctor's appointment in the afternoon with my doctor in Port St. Lucie. I rode over on my bike and as I usually did after a session with him, I went for a long ride. Sessions with the doctor were really hard. They did what therapists do best—get you to talk and cry and spill out all the junk you're going through! It was always emotionally hard on me. They were in actuality trying to save my life, but I would be affected for days and find myself retreating even more, isolating myself and somehow just getting by at school. My kids at school knew also that something was wrong. I told them about my blood disorder; and in every class there was a plan of action to save my life if all of a sudden my blood broke down and I started to spontaneous bleed. They just thought that was my problem—that I was worried over my blood disorder.

After visiting the doctor that afternoon, I found myself on the south side of Lake Okeechobee riding my bike and trying to settle down my troubled soul and spirit. I was traveling east on Route 80 when it began to get dark. After the darkness fell, I could see flashes of lightning off in the distance, so I stopped my bike and put on my rain gear over my riding gear.

I then got back on my bike and resumed riding. Everything seemed fine. There were no cars on that two lane highway either in front of me or behind me. It was clear sailing, or so I thought! Have you ever sat in your car at a stop light and seen it pouring rain on one side of the street, yet be perfectly dry on your side? That's exactly what happened to me, except it was dark and I didn't see it coming! I was doing the speed limit—65 mph, when I hit the wall of water unexpectedly. It was a virtual downpour! Not just a little rain shower! I have ridden many times in the rain before, but this was different. The moment I hit the wall of water I lost complete control of my bike.

Bikers know that when it first begins to rain, traction goes down to less than twenty percent. After thirty minutes traction goes back up to around eighty percent because it washes off many of the oils and the grease left on the road by different types of vehicles. That's why you see many bikers pulled off to the side of the road during the first few minutes of a hard rain.

My bike went down almost immediately. I hit the pavement head first at 65 mph! I saw "stars," little flashes of light in my brain, and then total darkness. But I was still somehow conscious (I think!), because all of a sudden I heard a voice as clear as a bell in my head speak to me. Remember now, I was feeling nothing and am totally surrounded by blackness. I heard the voice plainly and in a matter of fact way, tell me a set of instructions—When you come out of your roll, jump to your feet and move to the side of the road. There are two cars behind you. It all seemed perfectly normal and natural. I wasn't surprised or startled at all upon hearing the voice.

I then "felt" myself coming out of a roll and did exactly as the voice said. I jumped to my feet and moved to the side of the road. No sooner had I done that when a pickup truck, followed by a car, went around my bike, which was lying in the middle of the lane I had been traveling in and traveled directly over the spot on the highway I would have been lying had I not gotten up! All this took place in a matter of seconds. I felt nothing physically wrong at the moment and was very clear headed at the same time.

The two vehicles did not even slow down! They were traveling at a high rate of speed and continued on! I ran over to my bike to try to get it out of the highway before anyone else came through and hit it, causing another accident. I tried to pick it up, and that's when I realized something was wrong with my left hand. It didn't hurt. I just had no strength in it at all. I tried dragging the bike with my right hand and managed to get it turned slightly, but I couldn't move it.

Several more cars came and slowed down long enough to go around, but none stopped to help me. Finally a man and his girlfriend stopped and asked if I needed help. He helped me drag my bike into the ditch off of the road and then helped me gather up the debris from the accident. He let me use his cell phone to call Linda and then took me to Moorehaven and dropped me off at the Burger King. There Linda and a friend picked me up about an hour and a half later and took me straight to the emergency room in Okeechobee. Other friends from the church came with a trailer, located my bike, and took it home. The whole time it was still pouring rain.

God let me live. I hit the road headfirst at 65 mph! I've known people to die in a 10 mph crash while on a motorcycle! He deserves all the honor, glory, and praise! I don't know why, but I received only minor injuries from the crash. I had a cut beside my right eye from when my helmet hit the pavement and caused my visor to somehow pop in and cut me. It required six stitches. I also had two small bones broken on the top of my hand and a slight fracture of my wrist. None of those were actually even discovered until six weeks later! I had absolutely no road rash anywhere on me! Yes, I was sore for a few days, but that was nothing considering the crash I had had!

And what about "the voice"?! I know that the voice I had heard was God and/or my guardian angel saving my life. During the time I "blacked out" during the accident, it seemed like everything was in slow motion—the time, the voice, feeling myself come out of the roll (which I didn't know I was in!), jumping up and moving to the side of the road. It was all like a dream! But it was God! He knew exactly how many cars were there behind me. I didn't. I hadn't even seen them. Normally a person in an accident would just stay where he had landed for a moment collecting his thoughts and then finally get up if he could! But God moved my body to do what it needed in order to save my life!

That was on a Tuesday night. I missed school the next two days and then finally returned back to work on Friday. That's when another amazing thing happened.

Chapter 8

I returned to school on that Friday, three days after the accident. Several of our classes were combined in the auditorium to watch a film dealing with some sort of teen issue, when one of my students walked up to me. Juan is not a very talkative young man. He rarely says anything in class, but he is an excellent student and always respectful and polite to me. Up to that point he hadn't spoke three complete sentences in the month that school had been in session.

I was standing by myself at the back of the auditorium, when Juan got up quietly from where he was seated and walked back to where I was standing. He looked at me and said, "I understand you were in a bad motorcycle accident this week, Mr. Robertson."

I said, "Yes, Juan, I was."

He then asked, "Do you know why you survived the accident?" It was a rhetorical question, because he immediate answered it himself and said, "The reason you survived your accident is because God isn't finished with you yet. He still has a plan for your life." Then without another word he turned and went back to his seat.

I was stunned! I got goose bumps all over me and had to turn away in order to hold back the tears that were forming in my eyes! Talk about out of the mouths of babes! God had just sent a fifteen year old boy to me to let me know He still loved me and wasn't finished with me yet! You see, I was feeling as low at that moment as a person can feel! I was still sore from the crash; but even more, I was defeated in my personal life.

It was during the time just prior to the accident that I had begun texting and, on occasion, talking to people on my phone all over the state, both men and women, whom I had met through my attending motorcycle events and car shows, as well as through the internet. The night of my accident, Linda had found my phone and had gone through it, finding conversations I was embarrassed for her to see. I had reached out to people other than her in my pain. No, nothing was going on other than conversations, but they were not the persons I needed to be conversing with and have helping me with my pain and depression. She was heartbroken and angry.

Let me stop here and explain something. When I try to explain that my problem was depression, it seems so simplistic, because most people picture sadness, a detached state, or even a deeper hurting. My own negativity involved Satan's constant barrage of accusations and ugly ideas about myself, my family, and my wife, making me think that everyone was against me, that no one had ever really loved me, that they only used me and controlled me.

Satan knows our weaknesses, and when we are down, he adds fuel to the fire, building a negative picture where you feel that your life (no matter what it consists of) is useless, empty, and devoid of joy. Not everyone does blame others, but in my long time of loneliness, I blamed everyone I knew, especially my wife. For some reason I bought into the lie; and before long, I actually believed that my loving wife was the opposite of what she really is. I didn't want to be around her or anyone, most of the time.

Most people didn't understand, but it didn't ruin their lives. My wife was deeply hurt and devastated by it all (of course); and nothing she said made it better, because, as I found out later, it wasn't her—it was me, along with the depression and negative thoughts. I began to be deceitful with her, just for the heck of it. I would tell her I was going somewhere and then go somewhere else. I would tell her that I would be home at a certain time and then never show up or call. As hard as this is to admit, when she cried or got angry about it, I didn't even care. In fact, that pretty much described how I began to feel all the time about everything. I just didn't care anymore! I had sunk so low in my pain and hurt that all I could think of was self-survival! These other people were a distraction to keep me from having to deal with and battle the pain.

My doctors kept warning me about this, but I wouldn't listen to them either. They said that I would get to the point that

I didn't care about myself, as well, that I eventually would take my own life. But for some reason, I disregarded their warnings.

I also thought, in my unreasonable, self-seeking state, that I would like to converse with and get to know new people who had more in common with me than my so-called friends and my wife, who I felt just didn't get me anymore. Maybe they would understand what I was going through! They were interested in motorcycles or cars, and I could get dozens of calls a day or at all hours of the night to discuss stuff. I had never even met these people! I wanted to keep all this a secret from my wife because I knew she would never understand, and I didn't want her to give her opinion about it anyway!

Remember, I was angry and unreasonable most of the time when I was at home, which was becoming less often. At home, I had to face Linda, who really loved me and couldn't understand my pain and unhappiness. Away from home, I could play a game where I diverted my attention to all kinds of things and ideas and even people who had nothing to do with my real life.

My real life, I couldn't deal with, so I made up a new one, where I was always right, a long-haired, cool motorcycle guy who could talk to people, could go where I pleased, whenever I pleased, with no one to answer to—ever. So I played the game. I couldn't talk to my own wife much of the time. That was too painful. She wanted me to come home and straighten up—to be her husband. I could, however, find time to talk to others about nothing—the only topic I could handle.

I convinced myself that this was okay. What was her problem, I asked? My behavior caused so much grief in our relationship and almost cost me my marriage in the end. But Satan knew that all along, little-by-little, one bad choice after another, I was headed for a dead-end on a long and dangerous road.

Chapter 9

The accident shook me up in many ways. At this point I began reaching out to Linda and my doctors in earnest. I confessed my actions to the Lord and sought His forgiveness and then really sought to begin the healing with Linda. It was a wake-up call from God.

Two weeks after the incident, a neighbor of mine stopped by the house one morning. Linda and I have known him and his family for eighteen years, and our children have always been the best of friends. He is a good Catholic man who obviously loves the Lord. Though his practices and theology may differ from mine, over the years I have come to respect him very much because of his commitment to God, his church, and his family. He stopped and told me that the Lord had given him a "message" for me. He explained that he had a dream the night before in which the Lord had said that the incident with my motorcycle was not an accident—it was a warning! He asked me if I knew what it all meant. I said yes, but I didn't share with him, at that time, what I knew God was trying to tell me. Immediately, it came to my heart what God was telling me. Even though I was in the midst of a battle for my very life with my depression and bipolar disorder, I was still a servant of the King and was anointed and called by Him to preach the Gospel. Because of this, He would discipline me again severely the next time I allowed myself to go very far in my rebellious actions.

This series of events put me on a path of seeking help like I had never sought before. My pain, my anxiety attacks, my sadness, all had helped to cloud my reasoning and brought me to a place where I needed something to jar me! I tried. I really, really tried! I stepped back from the church again—indefinitely—to focus on getting well. I started staying home instead of being over at my mom's place as often or taking long rides on my motorcycle or in my car. I concentrated on taking my medications and trying new ones that were even stronger. It wasn't easy; I don't like taking medications—who does?

I still suffered greatly from anxiety attacks and extreme sadness. I felt constantly as if there were an elephant sitting on my chest! My mood swings were still hard to control. I was trying with every bit of strength I had! But it would eventually end up getting the best of me again. There was one more major incident in my life that would catapult me to depths I had never known before. Remember, I was battling both severe clinical depression and bipolar at the same time and trying to adjust to a medical condition that could end my life at any moment.

Let me remind you again of what "clinical depression" and "bipolar" disease consist of. This next series of paragraphs are from the University Medical Services out of Berkeley, California.

> *Clinical depression is a serious medical illness that negatively affects how you feel, the way you think and how you act. Individuals with clinical depression are unable to function as they used to. Often they have lost interest in activities that were once enjoyable to them, and feel sad and hopeless for extended periods of time. Clinical depression is not the same as feeling sad or depressed for a few days and then feeling better. It can affect your body, mood, thoughts, and behavior. It can change your eating habits, how you feel and think, your ability to work and study, and how you interact with people. People who suffer from clinical depression often report that they "don't feel like themselves anymore."*
>
> *Clinical depression is not a sign of personal weakness, or a condition that can be willed away. Clinically depressed people cannot "pull themselves together" and get better. In fact, clinical depression often interferes with a person's ability or wish to get help.*

Clinical depression is a serious illness that lasts for weeks, months and sometimes years. It may even influence someone to contemplate or attempt suicide.

People of all ages, genders, ethnicities, cultures, and religions can suffer from clinical depression. Each year it affects over 17 million American men and women (source: American Psychiatric Association). While clinical depression is common, it is frequently unrecognized and untreated.

In the same article from Berkeley is an explanation of Bipolar Disorder.

Bipolar disorder is characterized by cycling mood changes: severe highs (mania) and severe lows (depression). Sometimes the mood switches are dramatic and rapid, but most often are gradual. When in the depressed cycle, an individual can have any of the symptoms of a depressive disorder. When in the manic cycle, an individual is overly "up" or irritable. Someone in a manic state may appear excessively talkative and energetic, with little need for rest or sleep. This can affect thinking, judgment, and social behavior in ways that cause serious problems and embarrassment. For example, an individual in a manic phase may feel elated, full of grand schemes, or engage in reckless and /or other increased activities.

This was me—extreme lows, cycling mood changes, overly irritable at times, a need to get away, etc. Many, especially some in my own congregation, just thought I was weak and wanting an excuse to do whatever I wanted. They didn't understand, and many still don't to this day.

I had some even look me in the face and say I was trying to live out my second childhood or that I was going through a mid-life crisis! Some had been through some sort of depression themselves, so they judged me on whatever experience they were acquainted with.

I know many of them were praying for me, but few in the leadership team I had put together understood or even attempted to reach out to me on a personal level. On occasion I had to go to them in order to seek personal, hands-on prayer. Or, Linda would seek it for me. My music minister and her husband and my youth pastor and his wife were kind but also struggled with what to do with me. I had fallen off the pedestal.

When I look back at it now, I hold no ill will or blame over any of them. They just didn't have a clue. They were not trying to be mean or uncaring at the time; they had just not ever seen something like this before—especially in a minister. Ministers are put on a pedestal; and when they don't add up to what others think they should be, they lose respect and fall off the pedestal really fast! The accident had jarred me enough to seek serious help again. But it was just a matter of time before it would all blow up in my face once more!

Chapter 10

After my accident I began to be more consistent in taking my medication and trying to control the emotions that had been causing havoc in me for almost a year. The medications I was taking were much stronger than before, and I was now seeing my doctors as much as twice a week. I was out of church (preaching) indefinitely, but still attended. I was still trying to be a productive part of the ministry by encouraging with my words (calling) and my presence (visiting) as much as possible, both to those who were preaching in my absence and to the congregation as a whole.

On the outside it may have seemed that I was controlled and "with it," but on the inside I had sunk to a deep-seated sadness, which grew more and more each and every day. I was hurting—badly! It is hard to explain the feeling of complete sadness and a feeling of utter hopelessness, especially when there seems to be no apparent reason for it. This is how depression attacks you. I could barely function. I missed several days of school just trying to cope and not have the pressure of my job overwhelm me.

One day I was listening to a CD I have of a band called "3 Doors Down," a secular band. On the CD was a song that jumped out at me. In fact, I began to cry as I listened to it. It described exactly how I was feeling! I could never adequately describe how I was feeling to others before, but now I felt someone out there knew what I was going through!

Many times when I tried to tell others how I felt, all I would get was, "Oh, I've felt that way before"; and I knew full well they hadn't! It's like losing a close loved one and having someone who has never been through it say, "It'll get better. Just hang in there!"

I want to share the words of the song with you now so you can get a glimpse of what I was struggling with and what so many others are struggling with, even now as I write my story.

Away From The Sun
It's down to this, I've got to make this life make
sense
Can anyone tell what I've done
I miss the life, I miss the colors of the world
Can anyone tell where I am
'Cause now again I've found myself —So far
down, away from the sun
That shines into the darkest place
I'm so far down, away from the sun again—Away
from the sun again
I'm over this, I'm tired of living in the dark—Can
anyone see me down here
The feeling's gone. There's nothing left to lift me
up
Back into the world I've known
'Cause now again I've found myself—So far down,
away from the sun
That shines into the darkest place—I'm so far
down, away from the sun
That shines to light the way for me
To find my way back into the arms—That care
about the ones like me
I'm so far down, away from the sun again
(3 Doors Down)

I made several copies of the words to the song on paper, and
whenever anyone seemed to genuinely care what was going
on with me I would give them a copy of it and tell them to
find it on a CD and listen to it. This song was about depression! Someone out there knew what I was going through and
had described it in ways I never could!

Look closely at the words again: "I miss the life; I miss
the colors of the world. Can anyone tell where I am?" They
were right! The world no longer held any color for me! It
had come down to a matter of just trying to make it through
each day and then take a sleeping pill to get me through the

nights! I did feel I was so far down that the sun really wasn't shining anymore! I was in a deep pit that I couldn't climb out of!

"I'm over this, I'm tired of living in the dark

Can anyone see me down here

The feeling's gone. There's nothing left to lift me up

Back into the world I've known"

Feeling was gone! The ability to feel had been totally replaced by hopelessness and despair. Remember, depression is a mental illness. It is a chemical imbalance.

A person in severe depression cannot see the world as everyone else can. It is not the same as feeling sad or depressed for a few days and then feeling better. It affects every area of your life—your body, mood, thoughts, and behavior. It changes your eating habits, how you feel and think about things, your ability to work and study, and especially how you interact with people. I did feel as if I was "so far down, away from the sun" and those around me didn't care. They just wanted me to "get over it"! But I couldn't—I needed a miracle.

I really do appreciate my friends who tried everything they could to get me to "see" things differently. Our worship leader even took the time to go through every verse of the song and find a scripture that went with it, showing the promises of God, His abiding presence, and His healing power in our lives. But in all actuality, I needed James 5:14-16 to occur– "[14]Is any one of you sick? He should call the elders of the church to pray over him and anoint him with oil in the name of the Lord. [15]And the prayer offered in faith will make the sick person well; the Lord will raise him up. If he has sinned, he will be forgiven. [16]Therefore confess your sins to each other and pray for each other so that you may be healed. The prayer of a righteous man is powerful and effective." (NIV)

I believe in the power of prayer. I had taught our people to lay hands on the sick and pray. We had seen many miracles in our church as a result of claiming this particular verse.

Now I was the one that needed prayer. I don't blame them for their lack of understanding and compassion. I now know what the missing ingredient was—many lacked the baptism of the Holy Spirit and the subsequent faith and anointing it produces to walk in the power and anointing of the Spirit.

Unfortunately, no amount of positive reinforcement, kind words, or even God-inspired scripture could help me. For some reason, God was waiting for me to get to the complete bottom of the barrel and the end of myself, before He would break through the darkness and bring the healing I needed. I felt as if He had withdrawn from me, and the emptiness and grief just continually washed over me like a relentless ocean of pain. I understood this; I just couldn't do anything about it! I knew that God could heal me—whenever He wanted. He just didn't choose to do so until much later.

Chapter 11

After being out of the pulpit for almost two months, I came back in November. I preached the first three Sundays in November and even ordained two more men to be deacons that second Sunday. I was maintaining my balance, but just barely. That first Sunday in November I preached a message called "How Special We Are to God," and I used three points with scripture to show the congregation just how much God loves us. It was a message just as much for me as it was for them, because I wasn't feeling very special at the moment! In fact, I wasn't feeling much of anything other than deep sadness and despair. It was a message I had preached a year earlier, but from a little different perspective. Now, not only did I not feel special to God; in fact, I felt rejected and abandoned by Him!

That third Sunday in November I preached on "The Armor of God". My sermon was prophetic! I knew the scripture was true and that God's armor was for everyone, but I felt vulnerable to the onslaught of the enemy of my soul. My joy was gone; my life was wracked in despair and constant anxiety; and I had a deep sadness that nothing seemed to be able to eliminate. Even as I preached it, I felt weak, defenseless, and totally powerless. I was going through the motions, but I was sick and needing more help than either I or anyone else really realized.

The week after this, several misunderstandings with friends occurred and because of my heightened emotions and oversensitivity, minor situations that could have easily been cleared up, became life wrecking events in my mind. I was inconsolable and unable to be reasoned with about these misunderstandings. Even though my wife was on my side, I perceived that my whole life and career were going to be destroyed by these misunderstandings. I actually ran out of my house and down the road.

My wife went to the friends to try to clear things up, but I became panicky and anxious to the point where I couldn't talk to anyone or be reasoned with. They urged me to talk about it, but I couldn't. My emotions were all mixed up; I felt like I was going to explode and I had to run—again.

I got in my car and drove and drove, my tears blinding my eyes (seems crazy, huh?). I drove all night and all the next day. I went from the east coast of the state and then to the west coast trying to soothe the ache tearing me up inside. The doctor told me that being in my car was therapeutic for me. It was a way of self-medicating, because I could block out the rest of the world and turn everyone else off. He wasn't for it, but he understood it was my way of coping at the moment so I wouldn't have a complete meltdown.

I would pull off at rest stops or in parking lots to sleep— no one to bother me, no one to "misunderstand" me! I just wanted to be alone! My wife tried calling, texting, anything to get hold of me. She wanted me to go see my doctor, afraid I was finally over the edge and worried that I might inadvertently get in an accident or worse. That is the time the thoughts began to first come to me—thoughts of escaping my pain. I immediately threw them out, but they would return over and over again for the next two months.

She pleaded with me to go see my therapist. I knew I needed to. I was frantic! When I tried to talk on the phone to Linda, I was so upset and overly emotional that I hyperventilated and couldn't get the words out. I had to stop beside the road to try and pull myself together. "I believe in you," she kept saying. "Everything is going to be all right." "You are over-reacting." Again, I could see that I was over-reacting, but could not get myself together. My fears had overtaken me; the enemy was winning. Remember Satan comes to kill, steal, and destroy.

His goal was to steal my good friendships, my marriage, and my reputation, and to destroy any semblance of the decent life I had. Make no mistake, I know I made bad choices; but my ability to discern was so clouded and I became such a messed-up version of myself that no one really recognized me anymore.

Finally, the doctor called me, and I agreed to meet him in his office. He listened patiently to my account of what had happened (the misunderstanding with friends) and told me just what my wife had said. "This will blow over, nothing to go ballistic about. Calm down, everything will be fine." I knew that I had to calm down; every time I met with the doctor, I knew that if I did not get in control of my emotions, I risked being forcibly hospitalized. The doctor had already promised my wife that he would do just that if necessary.

The weird thing was that I would have times where I could discuss my church work, events coming up, etc. I could even, for a while, sit with my wife on our swing in the backyard and tell her that I loved her and didn't want this thing to be happening. I knew I was acting like a "wacko," but I couldn't figure out how to stop the cycle. Then, without warning, something would be said and I would perceive it as an attack; I would take off again, trying to run from whatever was chasing me down—something palpable. I could almost see it! Certainly I could feel that it was cold, angry, hurtful, accusing! The diagnosis was bipolar disorder, but I wonder how much was chemical and how much was spiritual warfare in all its insidious and destructive forms.

Then, the one thing I was clinging to in order to help me and give me stability was taken away, and I plunged into a pit, almost destroying my marriage for good and nearly losing my life.

Chapter 12

Let's pause for a moment, take a deep breath, and think about what has happened up until this point. Some of you are incredulous about some things that have happened in this story so far. I know! I would be, too! There's some stuff you don't understand. There are two things I want to mention.

First, several of you have commented to Linda and me on the fact that she was able to hang in there. How could she, because you sure wouldn't have! You're right: I'm just as amazed as you are—until I consider who God is and what amazing strength He gives us during difficult times.

There were many, even within our own family, who encouraged her to separate from me; but she wouldn't. I asked her to write down some of her thoughts and feelings. She wrote the following:

Even though at first, this whole mess seemed to be an unending, angry, and resentful episode from my husband, before long, I realized that there was more to it. Over the years my husband and I were best friends and that was the kind of marriage we had. When your best friend turns against you (that's what it felt like to me), you are devastated and confused.

He wasn't the person I knew anymore, but I kept seeing little glimpses of him from time to time; and I decided that if he were in a hospital, dying, I would never just walk out, so how could I do that now? Just because he hadn't been diagnosed with a physical disease did not make any difference.

I couldn't understand this deep darkness and I tried every way I knew to reassure him that God was still in control, but I am totally convinced that at times, I was dealing with something that had stolen my husband's life and was trying to take it from him. It was a real battle—mentally and emotionally.

*I prayed constantly; rarely did a night go by that
I didn't wake and pray intensely for long periods of
time throughout. After almost a year and a half, I
began to wonder if it would ever end. I had long conversations with God where He asked me what I was
going to do—if. Since I wasn't sure what my husband's frame of mind was, I thought he would very
likely leave me permanently or wind up dead somewhere because of his bad choices.*

*I finally decided that the only way for me to live
(without being submerged into the same pit of despair) was to do what God has always done for me—
totally forgive and take me back as His beloved.*

*I told God that even if there was nothing left of him
(my husband) except a thread of who he had been, I
wanted him back. I know that God can heal anything
if He just has one piece of us, alive, to work with.
Then I just waited and prayed.*

You might ask, Why did you put her through so much? If
you are still wondering that, then you still don't understand
depression; you are still thinking it is something that a person can control. I know this is true because several people
have told me since how they were able to just "get over it"
when they put their mind to it, that we know what we are
doing and can stop it. They were depressed, but they were
able to get out of it on their own and take responsibility for
their actions. That tells me they really don't know. Some
depression is temporary ("situational"), and some is much
more difficult and springs from chemical imbalances in the
brain ("clinical").

Each person's depression is different. Some depressions
are brought on by events and go away on their own. Others,
like mine, are life-threatening illnesses where your personality changes and you are not yourself anymore. It is awful for
everyone involved, and after a while you just can't take the

grief and heartache that has replaced your own feelings on a daily basis.

I do take responsibility for my actions, but I also know that I would have never done those things while in my right mind. I never did them before the depression, and I don't do them now after the depression. But, yes, I take responsibility and will also have to live with the consequences. Please don't think for a moment, however, that I was on a joy ride and looking for an excuse to do whatever I wanted. I was sick.

At this writing, over fourteen million people in the U.S. alone have been diagnosed with clinical depression. That is around 6.7% of the population of people eighteen years or older in any given year. Clinical depression is also the leading cause of disability in the U.S. for ages fifteen to forty-four. Friends, it is real; it is a disease, an illness that is due mostly to a chemical imbalance in the brain. It is an illness that can destroy family, tear down your health, and even eventually stamp out a life if gone undiagnosed and untreated.

The scary thing about it all is that it can happen to anyone! So, no, outside of God completely healing you through His miraculous power, you can't just "get over it"! Many will be on medication the rest of their lives. Some may get better through time with the help of medication and counseling and may even eventually not have to take any medication at all. Some may be healed directly by God's miraculous hand. But if you have true clinical depression, you don't just "get over it" on your own!

Second, in no way is my story meant to harm, injure, point fingers, or accuse anyone of injustices of any kind. This story is about me—and how God brought me through. Even though I will talk about certain situations and give some stories of interactions with other people, I have no hard feelings and in no way am I trying to hurt anyone. There are some things that were done by me and some things that were done to me that were just plain wrong, but I bear no ill will or unforgiveness. There are even some circumstances in which I have not only asked for forgiveness but also granted forgiveness to those who have hurt or offended me whether they asked for it or not. I learned a long time ago that everyone has a story. But this is my story. It is not my intention to bring harm or reproach to others through this. It is my story of events that shaped and defined who I am today.

You must understand something—I am a minister of the Gospel of Jesus Christ. I have pastored for many years and thus, have a pastor's heart. I am in the business of bringing healing and restoration to others, not tearing them down or trying to make someone look bad in order to justify a point or redeem myself in some way.

Does it mean that I agree with everything done to me or said to me during this time period? It doesn't. Does it mean that I am weak, a walkover, and people can treat me any way they want and say anything they want without my standing up for myself? No, but I will always try to bring reconciliation and healing to a situation, through the wisdom and grace of God. My having said all of that, let's go on to the next chapter!

Chapter 13

Thursday, December 4, 2008, was a day I will never forget. Linda and I had sat down to eat dinner that evening. Part way through she remarked to me that there was a meeting at the church that evening. She asked if I knew about it or remembered it. I told her that I had forgotten, so I quickly got up, got in my car, and went to the church. I went to the fellowship hall at the back of the education wing and sat down. The meeting was already in progress.

One of my associates was leading the meeting, and the group was just finishing up discussing "old business." He then announced they were now going to discuss "new business." Without any fanfare or emotion, he then said that he and four others of the leadership team had gotten together and decided they were going to ask me to resign as Senior Pastor of the church. He then said if I didn't resign, they would take me before the congregation and force me to resign. I was stunned!

Words cannot describe how I felt at that moment! It was the last thing I expected to hear! There was silence for a moment, and then he continued. He said that they felt I was too sick to continue. After a moment, I regained my composure and asked if instead of resigning, would they accept a leave of absence for three to six months, or even a year until I was better? He said no. It wasn't negotiable. They wanted me to leave. They didn't want to deal with my "sickness" anymore. He said they also wanted to go in a "new direction" with the church, and they wanted to get a new "lead" pastor. It was time for me to move on and time for the church to move on. He repeated that they didn't want to deal with my "sickness" anymore.

I then pointed out that out of the twelve people representing the leadership team and sitting there that night, I had appointed, hand picked, or ordained each one of them in the ministries they were filling. I talked about how I had been there for each one of them in both good and bad times. The answer was still no, and a cold hearted no, at that! I was heartbroken! I was totally devastated! I told the group that located in the foyer of the church, as you enter, is a picture of Jesus with the woman at the well. I said that we had always felt we were a church who reached out to people who were like the woman at the well—people no one else wanted, that we were a "woman at the well" church. We cared about people no one else cared about. I then told them that, now, I was the woman at the well, but Jesus was nowhere to be found in that group. At the time I needed them the most, they were going to throw me away like a piece of trash.

No one said a word. Most sat with their faces down. No one took up for me. I felt totally betrayed. I found out later from some of them that they were in a state of shock and were intimidated by the ones requesting this. Some were actually a part of the "overthrow" but were afraid to say anything about it. I then told them that this was a shameful day in the history of the church—shameful, shameful! Then I told them I would not resign, that they had better be prepared because the congregation would not tolerate this at all.

That is when the man next to me, one of the five men who were a part of this move to remove me, pointed his finger only inches from my nose and face, began to shake it at me, and began to loudly tell me over and over: "You are going to resign, you are going to resign. If you don't, we will force you to resign!" I told him that, no, I wasn't going to resign. He continued to shake his finger at me and yell at me that I was. He was very angry and aggressive. I was shocked and dismayed at this display of anger towards me. This is a man I loved as a brother and trusted to be there for me. I was devastated. I felt betrayed. Still no one intervened or even asked him to stop.

I got up from my chair and walked to the door. I then said, one more time, that I was not going to resign. He continued shaking his finger at me and yelling that I was going to resign, even as I turned and left and walked down the hallway.

I must confess that in my thirteen years of being in the church and pastoring that I have never encountered such gross disrespect for someone in a position of God given authority, such coldness and disregard. And the rest stood by without a word! I was in a state of shock. I was absolutely horrified and devastated over what had just occurred. My anxiety level was beginning to mount, and my depression and pain began to deepen as never before. I must add that this same man came to me two years later in deep repentance to God and ask for my forgiveness. He stated that during that time period that what he said and what he did were wrong. No excuses. He told me that he had failed me when I needed him the most. He was in tears, humble, broken, and contrite. Of course I forgave him. Restoration of relationships is the very heart of God!

I called Linda and discussed it with her. I finally decided I would resign. I felt that if we went before the congregation that I would certainly win, but at what cost? We would definitely lose the five families represented by those men, if not more. I did not start a church and raise it up for thirteen years, only to go through a church split. I decided I would walk away. We decided that it was best for the congregation to lose only two people, Linda and me, instead of possibly a dozen or more.

The magnitude of what had happened began to hit me. I felt rejected. I felt like I had just been thrown away like a piece of trash! I sank into a pit of despondency, which would plague me for two solid months. I also began to feel that Linda must have been involved in some way, that she had been instrumental in causing this horrible thing to happen. I called the church and left a message on the answering machine telling them that I would resign. I was angry and deeply hurt. I left and began to drive. I literally thought I was going to have a heart attack. These were people I loved and cared about—men and women I had raised up and trained!

I had only ever loved them, prayed for them, helped them through hard situations, given them opportunities to serve, only to have them throw me out as worthless. Where was their support when I needed it the most? Where were the men I had loved and prayed over, the men I had laid hands on and ordained, the men I had encouraged and given opportunities to minister? How could they turn on me in my deepest hour of need? I felt totally abandoned.

Some of you may ask, Why did you let this happen? Weren't you the pastor? It happened because I was sick. Had I been even a little healthier, I would have told each of them to get their things and leave, that they were being relieved of the positions I had appointed them to. I would have done a complete house cleaning and started from scratch, if need be. But I was sick. I thought they really loved me and would help me somehow get through the crisis I was going through in my life. I will talk about this in a later chapter when I tell what God revealed to me on why He allowed this to happen.

I have no anger or resentment over this now, and I have seen God work some great miracles in my life since; but at the time I was crushed. Needless to say, I couldn't work the next day. I left again—running, trying to soothe the pain I was in. I had not had a drink for over two months, but after this I became angry at God, angry at the men responsible, angry at those who had just sat there and did not take up for me; so I started drinking again.

I talked to Linda on the phone. I don't even know where I was at the time. She wanted to know if she could write a resignation letter for me. I told her to go ahead and write it and then sign it for me and give it to them. She did, and they read it that Sunday. Of course, I wasn't there. I was on the road again that Sunday morning, trying to drink the pain away in some parking lot in a town I don't even remember now.

There were many of those towns and many parking lots over the next two months. It was then that I decided to be completely by myself, so I moved a few of my things out and over to my mom's place. I had begun to blame Linda also and thought she was a part of the plan to have me removed. I was angry and resentful of her.

Most of December and January are a blur to me. I spent most of my time alone, holed up in my mom's trailer or in a bar somewhere on the coast trying to dull the edge. There were a couple of instances in the next two months where I wanted to just die. Linda was scared for me and called my psychiatrists on those occasions. They would call me and leave messages. Sometimes I would answer, and they would try to get me to come in and check myself into a facility before I harmed myself. I was so angry now, at the whole world! I vowed never to step foot in a church again!

Then on February the 5th, the pain was so intense that I decided to leave. I called Linda and told her that I wasn't coming back until God had done one of two things for me—He needed either to heal me or kill me! I wanted to die. I didn't care how—a heart attack or being hit by a Mack truck—it didn't matter. I just didn't want to hurt anymore.

Chapter 14

Starting back in December, a couple of members from the church, who came down each winter for the past several years, began to call me. John and Sandy would call and leave voice messages on my cell phone. They would always be encouraging and uplifting, never judgmental and condemning. They started out by saying things like, Dave, we'll be there in January. We can't wait to see you and Linda. We can't wait to see how God is going to heal you! We love you! Just little messages like that every few days or so.

My long time high school and college friend, Phil, would also call me and encourage me each week without fail. Linda continued leaving messages on my phone, both through voicemail and through texting. She would leave a message like, I love you. God is going to help us through this. He hasn't given up on you and neither have I!

I knew they were all praying for me. I knew that there were some faithful friends at the church also, who hadn't given up on me. I knew that they were interceding before God on my behalf for my healing and restoration. And they believed it would happen! I didn't. But they did.

Even with all this encouragement, I was not able to feel hopeful or good about anything. I was still living at my mom's house; and I still kept my wedding ring off, even though I knew both of these things hurt my wife and family. I couldn't stand to see her face when I would leave our home at night to go to my mom's house because I knew it hurt her so much. I was racked with guilt and pain, but my anger and resentment kept telling me not to trust her or anyone. I was on my own. These were all lies, but I couldn't see that at the time. My confidence in God had hit an all-time low; and I didn't feel worthy to come back to Him, even if He wanted me, which I was sure that He didn't.

After John and Sandy came down in January, Linda and I went over to their house several times, both together, on a good day, and on separate occasions. There I would cry and pour out my heart. I was broken and hurting and needed genuine friends desperately. I couldn't see that God had placed people in my life to help me get through this. I was blind. I couldn't stand what I saw in the mirror (even though I told my wife I liked the way I looked) and I couldn't stand the person I had become.

Throughout my life I had struggled with self-loathing, and it was now at a peak. I knew that many of the things I did were not healthy for me, but since I kept thinking that I was worthless, I couldn't believe that God or anyone else could or should still love me. Why should I waste time taking care of a piece of garbage? This was all a bunch of false thinking and lies from the pit of hell.

The frame of mind that had been crafted for me in my weak state was the same one that many people identify with—people I had once ministered to; and now I was the one who needed ministry. The problem was that I had developed these habits and ways of thinking that kept pulling me down. I would blame anyone who said anything that didn't agree with me. I wouldn't accept from anyone what I really needed. I was sinking fast in my hopeless state.

It was also during that time that I came face to face with something that I didn't really want to admit. I remember that we had taken my Dad out for his birthday on January 6th—Linda and I and my sister and her husband. My brother-in-law is in the counseling business and oversees many types of centers and facilities in another county. I was sitting across the table from him and asked him a question.

I said to him, "Is what I'm going through a severe clinical depression; is it a mental illness?"

I remember he looked me right in the eyes and said, "Yes, Dave, what you have is mental illness. You are mentally ill."

It hit me like a ton of bricks, and I began to cry. "Mentally ill" has such a negative connotation to those who don't understand it. Not long after that, I went to see one of my psychiatrists and asked him the same question. He had the same answer. He also said that until I came to grips with it, I would not get the help

I really needed. He had already spoken to me about what had happened with the church, saying it was terrible the way they had handled it. The traumatizing effect of that event had pushed me back at least six months to a year in the treatment process, but he wanted me to hang in there, keep taking my medication, and seriously think about admitting myself into a mental health facility for a couple of weeks to get back on track.

This was where I was at on February 5th. I had such intense pain that I didn't want to live anymore. I wanted to die. So I left. Then I began to drink, and drink, and drink. And yet at the same time I began to cry out to God to take away my pain and restore my life. It sounds crazy, doesn't it? But that is exactly what I did for three days.

On that Saturday, the 7th of February, I stayed in a rented place close to Brandon on Route 60 so I could spend the weekend drinking myself unconscious. I had been sleeping in a Walgreen's parking lot up until then, but decided to find a place where I could spend the rest of the weekend and drink myself unconscious. That Saturday I drank so much that I could barely function. I was practically in a fog. The pain was dulled. I had succeeded, but I was still alone and wanting my life back or wanting it over.

I remember that there were times during that day that I would cry out to God to hear me and to answer me. But I didn't feel as if my prayers went any further than the walls around me. For some reason (I didn't understand at the time) He kept His healing from me. I finally fell asleep totally wasted. I had been drinking all day. More than I can ever remember having drunk before.

I slept completely through the night and woke up around 8:00 a.m. When I got up, something seemed different. I couldn't place my finger on it at first, but something was different! It hadn't quite registered with me yet; all I knew was that when I woke up I had an intense desire to find my wife, hold her, and tell her I loved her. My heart was also light!

I knew Linda was going to church that day in Vero Beach at Central Assembly. Sandy had called me earlier on Friday and left a message saying that she and John were going to take Linda to church there, and asked me to join them. At the time I had no plans of going into any church! But this Sunday morning I had an overwhelming desire not only to see Linda, but to go to church! It still didn't strike me that something was different. I got a shower as quickly as possible, got dressed, and before I knew it, I was traveling east on Route 60 toward Vero Beach!

As I was driving, I found myself doing something I hadn't been able to do for a long time—I turned on a praise and worship CD and began singing with all my heart to the Lord! As I was singing, I began praising God. Tears began to trickle down my cheeks; and before I knew it, I was weeping before the Lord. I must have been quite a sight to those who passed me!

There I was—one hand on the wheel and the other lifted to the Lord in praise! I then began praying out loud and found myself repenting and glorifying God all at the same time. And then it hit me like a ton of bricks—I wasn't in pain anymore! I didn't have this elephant sitting on my chest; my depression was gone—Hallelujah! After a year and a half of hell on earth, I was free! Also astounding was that there wasn't a sign of any hangover at all!

Something was very different that morning, something amazing. The depression that had choked out my life and opened the door for so many terrible choices had been erased, like a bad dream! Did it really happen? It had, and it was gone! God had healed me! I began to rejoice even more. I could feel that the horrible and ugly mental pressure I had been under for so long had been replaced with a heart of praise to our Lord and Savior Jesus Christ. At that moment, I knew I wanted to receive from those who really cared. I cried; I prayed; I sang; and if I hadn't been in such a hurry to find my wife, I would have also stopped the car on the side of the road, got out, and danced!

I texted Linda and asked if I could meet up with them somewhere after church was over and go to lunch. She texted back to me that they would. I didn't tell her I was on my way to church. I had told her before that I would never go into any church again and had even felt resentment any time I had passed a church on the highway for the past two months. Now, I wanted to surprise her. I was actually excited and looking forward to something for the first time in a long, long time. I wanted her to see her "healed" and "free" husband with her own eyes!

When I got to church, it had already been going on for about twenty minutes. She was sitting at the back with John and Sandy and did not see me enter. I slipped in and there was an empty seat beside her (not an accident), so I sat down. When she turned around to see who was there, she was so surprised and happy! We grabbed each other and began crying. We expressed our love for each other, and I told her that God had healed me. Of course, John and Sandy were rejoicing with us!

After the service, Linda took me up front to meet Pastor Buddy Tipton. She told me that he had said to her that morning he wanted to meet me. When he saw Linda and me coming towards the front, he immediately broke away from the group he had been talking to and came over to us. He reached out to shake my hand, hugged me, and said he had wanted to meet me and was waiting for that opportunity. He said that God wanted him to work with me. Then he took us back to his office, where for almost an hour and a half, he cried with us, prayed with us, encouraged us, and ministered to us.

I must go back and recount something else that occurred that morning. When Linda, John, and Sandy arrived at the church that morning, Pastor Buddy met them at the door and introduced himself to them. Sandy just blurted out that Linda was in a crisis situation. Of course, God had already planned this whole thing out, but they didn't know it. Linda was nervous, but she briefly explained that her husband was a pastor who was in a terrible situation. He was hurting and so were many others because of it. That was all she said. He told her that he wanted to work with me. He asked for my phone number and said he would be glad to call me sometime. They didn't know that God had gotten me up and was steering my car to that very place.

In the meantime, John just felt that I might show up. He kept going outside to check for my car. So even as the service started, John continued looking over his shoulder, hoping that I would be there that morning. Sandy had told Linda earlier that she believed a miracle could happen that morning. Linda wanted that too, but was worn down by now and bracing for more disappointment.

Pastor Buddy had come by where she was sitting before the service and asked her to see him after church to explain more about the situation with me. He really didn't know anything at all about it, but wanted to help us and he let her know that.

Now understand, I had not been in church for two months. I had given no indication whatsoever that I was going to be there that day, or any other day, for that matter! And up until that morning I had no intention of ever going back into any church again! But for some reason, John seemed to know that God was going to bring me to church that day and bring healing and restoration back into my life. And why not!? He and Sandy had been praying fervently for me and had complete faith in what God was going to do!

Healing took place that day, but that was just the beginning of what God was going to do in my life through His amazing power and grace, the love and prayers of my wife who never gave up on me, friends who believed in me and in God's miracle power, the mentoring of a pastor who has become my personal friend and spiritual father, and the ministry of an incredible church family that loved on me and accepted me unconditionally. But that's not the end of the story.

Chapter 15

When I say God healed me, I mean it—"plain and simple." All signs and symptoms were eradicated. I had no lingering sadness or anger or emotional roller coasters. The mental illness was gone! In fact, about a month after this happened, both my medical doctor and my psychiatrist re-evaluated me. Their diagnosis was that a miracle had occurred! They both admitted that there was no other explanation.

My medical doctor said that many times doctors will try to explain things away in order to avoid an explanation that might justify the supernatural one, but that all doctors have witnessed miracles at some point in time and he wasn't going to deny that my healing was a miracle. Both of them released me from their care and from the use of any medications. They wrote me down as "cured"!

Two weeks after my healing, upon the suggestion of my pastor and my wife, I went to a ministry offered after the Sunday morning church service. It is called "Prophetic Ministries." This is where people with prophetic gifts use them to encourage and build up the rest of the local church body. I was very skeptical about what might be going on and what might be said, so I was a little nervous going in.

I knew that God gives gifts to His children at the time of their salvation, and I knew that many gifts were also given to those who asked, according to the New Testament. I was totally ignorant of this particular gift, however. Since then, I've researched it extensively in the Bible and found it to be one that we are all encouraged to seek (I will elaborate on this later). So I went in.

A lady led me to one of the Sunday School rooms and introduced me to three people who were sitting there before me. I did not know any of them, and they had no idea who I was. I had already asked Pastor Buddy two weeks earlier not to reveal who I was to anyone, and he was faithful to my request. I wanted to be incognito, to fly under the radar at this new church.

When I sat down, the man in the middle told me that they were going to pray for me first and ask God to reveal to them some things that would be an encouragement to me. They prayed for a few minutes, while I sat there getting a little nervous. Then I prayed quietly, also, and asked God to give me a word of direction and encouragement to help me back on the road to recovery from the year and a half of hell on earth I had just come through. I told the Lord that whatever He wanted to show me, I would listen.

Then the man in the middle looked up and asked the other two if they were ready. They both said yes, so he began. He told me that God had shown him a city with many buildings in it. In the middle of the city was a tall skyscraper standing high above the surrounding building. The skyscraper had a roof that was on hinges and it was in the process of opening. The roof was about halfway open, and out of it many bad and hurtful things were flying; but at the same time the light of Christ was flowing into the building with many blessings and good things. The light of Christ was refreshing and renewing me.

He said God had revealed to him that I was that skyscraper, that in the past I had been in ministry of some sort and as a result many souls had been saved. He said that the Lord told him to tell me that whatever ministry I had been involved in before, it was very small compared to the ministry I was going to have in the future and that many souls would be saved as a result of it. He added that the number of souls saved through my previous ministry would also be small compared to the number of souls who would come to Christ as a result of my new ministry! Then he looked at me quizzically.

I wondered how he knew I had been involved in ministry, how these people knew anything about me at all. They had no idea who I was! It was then that I knew God was speaking directly to me through this man! I was so overwhelmed by it all that I began to cry, but I didn't say anything. I cried because God revealed that He wasn't finished with me yet. Others (myself included) may have counted me as too messed up and may even have thrown me out, but God doesn't make junk. Where others see rubbish, God sees valuable and useful tools for His kingdom. He also cares that we feel that way, and He makes sure that He lets us know—through his Word, or through godly people—that He is not finished with us at all.

Then the leader said one more thing. He said God revealed to him that I was going to become good friends with and be mentored by a man who was a little taller than me, with short, light colored hair, and fair skin and that this man would play a significant role in my life. He didn't realize it at the time, but he had just described Pastor Buddy! This blew me away also, because Pastor Buddy had already begun mentoring me by taking me out to eat after each service, counseling with me, and calling me several times a week to check on me and encourage me.

Then the woman to my left spoke. She said God had revealed to her that I had been through a hard time over the last year, that I had been taken through the fire. She went on to say that first of all, there was no condemnation to those who are in Christ Jesus and that I was in Christ. Christ did not condemn me for the sins and mistakes I had made in the past. Second, God wanted me to know that I was totally forgiven and my trespasses were not held against me. They were under the Blood of Christ, never to be remembered against me again! I really began to cry then, but still offered no explanation to them about myself or spoke to them other than to say, "Thank you."

Then the man to my right began to speak. He said God had also revealed to him that I had been through a real hard time in the past year but that even though I was forgiven and there were those I had forgiven, there was one person I had not yet forgiven and needed to do so. Immediately I began to go over in my mind who that might be. I had earnestly sought the Lord for my own forgiveness for the things I had said and done during my illness. I had also forgiven those who had hurt me so deeply at the church. I just couldn't put my finger on who that might be! We will come back to this later, because, at a later event, I do recall who the person is; and in and of itself it is an incredible story. Who said the Christian life was a bore!

Then he told me one more thing that blew my mind—he said that the Lord told him to tell me that the sermon Pastor Buddy preached that day was specifically for me, that even though the rest of the congregation would benefit from it, it was specifically a message from the Lord to me. I really began to cry then! The message Pastor preached that day was about how we are the righteousness of God in Christ Jesus. It says that when God sees us, he sees us as holy and righteous before Him, not based on anything we have done, but simply on what Christ has done by shedding His own blood for us and then clothing us in His own righteousness!

You see, I was carrying a lot of guilt at the time. Even though I had preached messages similar to this myself, I believed it for others, but always had a hard time believing it for myself. At this time of my life I was really feeling unworthy. I felt I had let my wife down, let my family and friends down, let my church down, and ultimately let God down. But God was letting me know in my brokenness that He did not see any of those things, that others may hold them against you, but God sees you through the precious blood of Jesus. I wept like a baby. I'm not ashamed to say it. Not only was I healed, I was forgiven!

Then they prayed over me before I left. I had not spoken anything to them other than to thank them. I left the room and started back through the church, which was empty by this time. A woman came through the back door and asked if my name was Dave. I told her yes. She said that I was to meet Pastor Buddy, his wife, and Linda in his office, that he was going to take me to lunch. So I made my way back to his office.

When I stepped through the door, the three of them looked at me with big grins on their faces and said, "Well?!" So I began recounting what had been told to me. They laughed and they cried with me about it; and then when I got to the part about the message, they all began to just laugh and laugh. I said, "What is it?" Pastor Buddy then said that just before I had walked in the door, he was telling them that after he had spoken to me on Wednesday, after church service, God had laid on his heart a message and that it was a message God had given to him for me, even though the whole church could benefit from it; and that's what he preached that day!

Needless to say, I was both awestruck and rejoicing at the same time! God spoke though one man and then verified it through the other! Pastor had not spoken to anyone about me at all, or about why he preached that message that day. God was letting me know, beyond a shadow of a doubt, that He had spoken directly to me through the words of others!

A few weeks later, the lady who had ministered to me that day came to me after a Sunday evening service and said she needed to tell me something that she hadn't been able to share before. She said that when I came into the room that day, she and the other two men saw and felt God's anointing and glory all around me. They didn't have any idea who I was, but they saw I had God's special hand upon me. After I left, she said they all turned and looked at each other and asked, "Who was that masked man?" Someone said, "God's anointing is all over him!" and they wondered who I was.

Again, I was dumbstruck about it and so proceeded to ask Pastor Buddy about it. He explained to me that even though I had been through a hard time, the Bible says: "For the gifts and callings of God are irrevocable." (Romans 11:28; New King James Version). In other words, God doesn't change His mind. His calling on my life to preach the Gospel hasn't changed one little bit just because I went through an illness and made some bad choices along the way. I was forgiven and His call on my life was just as real now as it ever was!

When He calls us to do something and anoints us with that calling, He never takes it back. Once you've been called into ministry, you will always be a minister. The circumstances may change, but the calling stays the same. That was why they sensed God's anointing around me because I am still a minister under Christ and His call and anointing are just as valid today as they were when He first called me. That was good news to me.

Two weeks later I went to a "Men's Encounter" through the church with fifty other guys. You won't believe what happened there!

Chapter 16

How many of you know that we accumulate a lot of junk along the way as we travel this path of life? It starts out when we are children and threads its way into many areas of our lives, even up to the present. Sometimes it is even handed down to us as generational curses. The Bible speaks of these things.

I know in my own life that the seeds for depression were planted in me many years ago, even as a child. Satan knows that also, and he is waiting for just the right moment to pounce and bring destruction into our lives. He has come to kill, steal, and destroy the good things God has planned for us.

Four weeks after my initial healing and two weeks after my incredible encounter with the Prophetic Ministries team, the church paid for and sponsored me as a participant at their "Men's Encounter." I didn't know what to expect. Boy, what a surprise I received! As a minister, I have been to all sorts of seminars; special training; classes, including Promise Keepers; and leadership training and development. I have also been in charge of and taught different types of classes and leadership training programs. But I have never before encountered what I did that weekend.

This was a time of getting one on one with God, both individually and in a corporate setting. I went in healed of my depression and bi-polar condition, but still wounded, hurting, and feeling terribly rejected by my church and others. I also was in deep sorrow over how I had acted during the time I went through my illness.

I knew the whispers were out there. I knew that some were skeptical of what God had done in my life and that others were spreading gossip as if it were God's truth. Eventually, it all gets back to you, and it hurts. I also knew that I had some issues in my past that I wanted resolved and was totally open to the Spirit of God bringing those issues to light and helping me to deal with them. That was the background for the encounter.

I won't reveal how the whole thing went, but I want to share with you one instance during that time, when I received complete freedom. During the encounter, a young man from our church led us in praise and worship before each session. The song that stood out for me over and over was "Mighty to Save." These words resonated in my spirit each time I heard them; but they would mean more to me later, after the encounter was over.

I had the good fortune of being paired up in a room with another participant, who, I eventually learned, had also gone through depression. Wow! Someone who understood what I had gone through would be my roommate for the next couple of days. God knows what he is doing! I still did not reveal to anyone that I was a minister. I wanted to be treated just like everyone else. I still did not feel worthy enough to carry that designation.

I was put in a group of six men, two of them being the leaders of that particular group. The leader of my group, Richard, was a very kind and loving gentleman, who was a little older than me. On that Saturday afternoon, during one of our large group sessions, one of the leaders gave his testimony and then went into a teaching on forgiveness. Not only did he talk about God's forgiveness for us, but also that we should forgive others just as Christ forgave us. I sat there and thought to myself, This session has nothing to do with me at all! I know all this stuff! I had preached and taught about it myself many times in the past. How wrong I was!

At the end of the session, all the group leaders came forward and stood at the front to receive anyone who wanted to pray. Almost every man went forward to pray with someone, except for me. There was a tremendous time of victory in many lives that afternoon, but I still sat there, in the back row, believing I was not needing any help at the moment.

Then, all of a sudden, one of the other leaders got up and asked for the microphone. He said that God had revealed to him that there was still someone in the group who needed to come forward to pray. He said God had shown him someone in a vehicle traveling along. Then the vehicle stopped and this person got out. The vehicle then continued on without him. The Lord showed him that this person is not forgiving someone.

As he talked, I was thinking to myself, He's definitely not talking about me! He's talking about someone that has to do with some car or something." Then he continued and said that in the prophetic, a vehicle usually meant a type of ministry and that someone in the room had been in ministry of some kind, but then had to leave it. He said that there was someone the person needed to forgive!

I was in shock! The moment he completed his sentence, the convicting power of the Holy Spirit hit me like a ton of bricks. I immediately leaped to my feet and practically ran to the front.

I went up to Richard, my group leader, and began to literally sob on his shoulder. He hugged me and asked what it was that I needed to pray about. I continued to just sob and sob. I could barely get the words out. I told him that they were talking about me! I was the one! I was the one in the ministry! He asked me if I had any unforgiveness towards anyone. I told him that I thought I had forgiven everyone. Then I told him some of what I had been through in the past year. That's when he asked me another question, "Have you forgiven yourself?"

Immediately the Holy Spirit spoke into my heart and showed me—it was me! I had forgiven every one else, but I couldn't forgive myself. I had been healed, but I was still punishing myself for the year and a half I had been sick. I couldn't forgive myself because I knew I had hurt my wife so deeply. I also felt as if I had let my congregation down. So I began to pray and cry out to God. I asked Him to forgive me and release me from that burden, which was a heavy one. He had forgiven me, and I had forgiven others; but I had not forgiven the one person that really needed to be set free— me. God was faithful. When I released that year and a half to

Him, the guilt lifted like a feather. I walked away from that session a free man.

I mentioned a song earlier that had great impact on me, starting with the Men's Encounter. The song is called "Mighty to Save." The words of that song resonate deep within my spirit. Most of the time when we sing it at church, I cannot hold back the tears. Look at the lyrics to this song and you will see why this has such an impact on me.

Mighty to Save

Everyone needs compassion, Love that's never failing;
*   Let mercy fall on me.*
Everyone needs forgiveness, The kindness of a Sav-
*   iour; The Hope of nations.*

Saviour, He can move the mountains,
My God is Mighty to save, He is Mighty to save!
Forever, Author of salvation.
He rose and conquered the grave, Jesus conquered the
*   grave!*

So take me as You find me, All my fears and failures,
*   Fill my life again.*
I give my life to follow, Everything I believe in, Now I
*   surrender.*

My Saviour, He can move the mountains,
My God is Mighty to save, He is Mighty to save!
Forever, Author of salvation,
He rose and conquered the grave, Jesus conquered the
*   grave!*

Shine your light and let the whole world see,
We're singing for the glory of the risen King . . .
*   Jesus (x2)*

My Saviour, He can move the mountains,
My God is Mighty to save, He is Mighty to save!
Forever, Author of salvation,
He rose and conquered the grave,
Jesus conquered the grave!

My Saviour, you can move the mountains,
You are mighty to save, You are mighty to save!

Forever, Author of Salvation, You rose and conquered
    the grave,
Yes you conquered the grave!
                    (Hillsong Australia)

Yes, I needed compassion, love that never fails, and mercy; and I found it in the arms of Jesus!

Yes, I needed forgiveness, the kindness of a Savior, and hope; and I found it at the foot of the cross!

Saviour, He can move the mountains. He did what no doctor could do for me: He completely moved the mountain of depression and set me free! He was (and is) mighty to save! Hallelujah!

He did take me as He found me, with all my fears and failures and filled my life again!

Now I do give my life to follow. Everything I believe in; and now I have completely surrendered to the will of God in my life!

Why can He move the mountains in our lives ? . . . because He died and rose again, conquering sin, death, and the grave!

I am going to shine my light so the whole world can see. I will sing for the glory of the King of kings!

Everyone has a story. This is mine. What is yours?

Where are you in your walk with Christ at this very moment? Whatever situation you find yourself in, He can move the mountains. Whatever He has called you to do, He will be faithful to fulfill it in you through His strength.

God can do a miracle in your life, also. Sometimes He chooses to intervene without doctors, but many times He puts the resources around us to use, such as doctors and medications. Whatever way He chooses, there are valuable lessons to be learned for each of us, and then it is our responsibility to share the lessons and knowledge we have gained from the experience in order to help and encourage others around us.

You might be running from God in your pain as I did. If so, are you done running? Are you at the end of what the world can do for you? Are you at the end of yourself? When we are at our weakest, with nowhere left to turn, that's when He can save us from the mess we've made of it all. He has the all the answers and He's the only one who does.

Maybe there is someone you know who is going through a rough time with depression right now. If so, maybe my story can encourage them to believe that there is someone out there who understands exactly what they are going through. Do you remember the morning I was healed? As I was traveling in my car and praising God, a scripture kept coming to me over and over again. I want to share it with you as I close out Part 1 of my story: Psalm 118:5—"In my distress I prayed to the Lord, and the Lord answered me and set me free!"

To God be all the glory, honor, and praise!

Part 2

MY
PATH OF
HEALING

(Linda's Story)

Chapter 17

What do you call a process that feels as if it is going to kill you, squash out every bit of life in you, and turn you into a big lump of pain? Do you call it growing? I don't. Do you call it trial by fire? That's a little better, but still not there. When I look at the whole thing, shake it out and examine it, I want to call it my "path of healing." A path is a way and healing is returning something that has been hurt or broken to a condition as good as it was before or better. It doesn't hurt anymore; in fact, you can touch it, think about it, talk about it, and examine it. Nope, it doesn't hurt. A miracle and divine intervention are the only explanation.

How can that be? Well, first of all, let me say something you may already know. Nothing is really what it seems to be, at first. Life is a lot more complicated than that. We are a lot more complicated than that. When God put us together, he did a real work of artful crafting. He fashioned so many beautiful feelings and ideas into a human body that was going to be flawed. The human soul would be so desperately lost without Him. The human experience is so full of potential for godliness and, at the same time, of propensity for sin. We are all like that. No one is different. We are all the same. We all need redemption and forgiveness.

But we all want our heroes to be different. We want our husbands and fathers to be the ones who defy the odds. Somehow, we think they are a cut above the rest. When they aren't, because they can't be, it's somehow devastating, even though we know ourselves that we are just like every Adam and Eve person that ever lived. Yes, we are full of mistakes or boo boos, misjudgments or whatever. But not my "knight in shining armor, the one true good man left on the planet.

Well, just get your head out of the clouds, Cinderella! Prince Charming is a fairy-tale, and you don't want or need a paper guy. You need a real man. It's just that you cling so hard to what "ought to be" that you sometimes forget what reality and God's word says. "All are sinners; all have fallen short of God's best plan." All means all, sister; think about it.

That's how I pictured my husband. I know he has many faults, and I have been the first one to point them out. But I really always thought that some things that affected other people would never be able to touch us because, well, he was just too "with-it" for that. I had long ago stopped worrying what to do when he made little mistakes. Of course I would do the standard: 1) Bring the mistake to his attention. 2) Repeat #1 as often as needed! This was my habit. God would prove me right over a period of time and that would be that—or so I thought.

We might disagree over little things, but not often; and he usually decided to make me happy because it really didn't matter what happened over most issues. He wanted to make his wife happy, and isn't that the goal of all good husbands?

I know this sounds silly, but ask my friends—my husband loved me and everything about me. He was just happy to be in this thing and so was I. We enjoyed our children (we both had them when we got married). We had our differences over the discipline of them, but we got through that, as well. For sixteen years, our life seemed so very full of busy church work, busy family times, and busy school life. We were both school teachers, as well as parents, (kids now grown and on their own), grandparents (four beautiful grandchildren) and both of us were devoted to the people of our church (our ministry) where Dave pastored.

So how did this train wreck (the depression) happen? How did I go to sleep one night married to Prince Charming and wake up the next morning married to a stranger who didn't want anything to do with me and frankly acted like I was a pain in his butt? Of course it didn't happen overnight, but I didn't see the severity of it. I knew he was increasingly unhappy and tired.

He was seemingly sick or hurting somewhere in his body all the time. But I had no idea he was on the edge of a full blown melt-down—not my husband.

I'm telling you, he would go to bed at 11:00 wake up at 3:00, read his Bible, pray, write a sermon, make a Power-Point to accompany it with awesome graphics, text, and pictures, go back to bed at 5:00, and get up at 6:30 bright-eyed and full of enthusiasm. He taught school five days a week; planned sermons and teachings for Bible studies; handled administration for the growing church; hired people to help; and counseled, married, and buried people. For many years he also planned and led the music after learning to play the guitar from scratch. One year from when he started the praise-team music, he was teaching others at churches in our area how to do the same thing. I'm not kidding—he really did all this!

He called those who were discouraged and down and delighted in baptizing and preaching. He did funerals and memorials with video tributes he had made himself with photos from loved ones. He did this for years. I got used to it. Must be God-energized, I thought (like the energizer bunny only from heaven instead!) No human alone could keep up this schedule, I reasoned.

He also planned elaborate training programs and materials, as well as reports, devotions, and programs for the church—all to perfection. It was truly the work of several people (several really talented people!)

I just gave up trying to figure out how he managed it. I just took it for granted that he would always be like that. It was fun to be around all that and exciting, too. I had a part in everything. We enjoyed doing all this together. We knew God had called us for it—it was natural. People came to the church who did not like church. They came because they felt loved and accepted, and in addition, he was an excellent preacher. They wanted to hear and know more. It was great. We gave up any time that we could for this cause. We were available anytime of the day or night for our congregation. We were glad to do it.

At the same time, my hero could teach the socks off anybody I ever heard in the classroom. I'm not kidding. He taught high school kids and loved it (still does). On occasion, I would pop in his class to see what was up and was always amazed at the wonderful things going on. I am a teacher, too, and so I spent a little free time in his class. He taught his heart out for those kids, and they always loved and respected him. I loved listening to him teach; he was interesting. I told him he was the best teacher I'd ever heard, but I don't think he really believed me. Whenever we saw his students anywhere in town, they would get all excited and shake his hand or hug him and would you believe that he always remembered their names!? How he did it I don't know.

Anyway, when you think of this superachieving man of God and then you see him crash head on into an invisible wall, you gasp and step back. What a terrible thing, you think. What did he do wrong? He must have done something wrong to deserve this awful curse on his life. You look for an easy answer. You look for the obvious. You examine the whole thing and then you shake your head. But what if you had to experience it yourself? When the person crashing is the other half of your body, you crash too. You have had on a blindfold; and when the blindfold comes off, you see the part of your body you thought was invincible, lying on the ground in a pile of broken bones. He can't get up; you can't help him up; no one can help him up. You cry out to God, you wait, you cry, you wait—on and on.

Chapter 18

At first Dave would complain a lot. That didn't do him any good. I felt that he had a big problem. He did, but so did I! He was unhappy with only two things—everything I said and everything I did. How did that happen? It was like he had PMS all the time. It was a bummer! I tried to remain upbeat, but it was hard. "You are boring," he said once. What, are you kidding me? I thought. I just laughed even though it hurt my feelings. Then I got mad and he left. I made a list of all the "unboring" things I do. Do you remember when I said that things are not always what they seem? He was trying to shake off his sad feelings, but I didn't recognize it.

He tried to figure out a way to get rid of the pain. He really was in pain, emotional pain; I could see that, but I didn't know why. I was mostly angry at him for being so messed up. I would tell him over and over about all the things he had going for him. He had a wonderful life, fabulous family (all healthy), great job at school, a growing ministry with the church, a home, and many other things that others only wish for. Nothing cheered him up.

Believe me; I tried thinking of everything I could. I am a self-taught psychoanalyst (just kidding—all wives are), so I began to take this thing apart piece by piece. I tried to figure out what was wrong, but I couldn't understand how or why he just couldn't get out of it. I began watching every move he made, trying to figure out what was going to happen next. That didn't work. Those bipolar episodes kicked in; and like I said, it was like he would just go off the deep end about little things and not be able to level out again.

Maybe you can identify with this if you have ever had PMS or been around someone with it (hasn't everybody?). It's a chemical imbalance that affects women once a month, and it can be pretty unsettling. I have had a few bouts with it myself, so I started thinking on those terms. Bipolar seems to be a lot more gripping than PMS, however, because I could always come back to my normal level of thinking in a day or

70

so; and I even kept a calendar, for years, to help me deal with the mood swings that would come.

I would think, Okay, is this situation really aggravating me, or am I getting into that time of the month when I can't think straight? If it was that "danger zone" time, I would bite my lip and just try to avoid talking altogether, because something ugly could definitely come out! The problem was that when he got into an episode, he stayed there: he was irritating, not nice, and grouchy, and he sometimes made mean comments. Hey, I don't think I like you anymore, fella! Even though I loved him, I sure didn't like him at all at that point!

I had been praying for him for over a year to get healing for all those hurting places he complained about. Also, it just seemed he was never satisfied with anything. He had so many unreasonable expectations of himself (I thought). "You just can't be perfect all the time," I would say. I wanted him to be really happy, not just glad for everyone else or just glad to be existing. I know that God wants us to have peace and happiness in our lives, daily. He loves us. He's our father, and we want that for our kids, right?

Well, anyway, I would pray for Dave to get healing for all of it. I believe that prayer is the answer for just about everything because we are trusting in God, not ourselves, to take care of the situation. The only problem is that you don't know when or how the answers will come. It can get pretty tedious waiting. And in this situation, it got awful, a lot more awful, before it got better.

It seems like Dave had to go through all of these "stages" of dealing with his depression before he could get to a place where God came into it. I went through "stages" too. A lot of them were not pretty—wait a minute, none of them were! It was just pure misery . . . .

Chapter 19

The first stage of the depression was sadness and lack of enthusiasm about anything. It went on for quite a while before the second stage kicked in

The second stage of the depression that I noticed was irritation. I have already talked about it. He was irritated and then I was irritated that he could possibly be irritated when he was so obviously blessed! I tried to let this go, because I still thought that this would soon pass. In the meantime, Dave told me that he was having anxiety attacks and felt nervous constantly.

An anxiety attack is a panicky "gotta-run-from-this-place" feeling in the pit of your belly. It's scary, so fear and panic are both in there. That made no sense to me whatever. How could you just be sitting there watching TV and suddenly feel like running away in the next minute? However, he kept telling me the same thing. Eventually, he did get up and drive around, alone, in his car. I didn't like this at all. Why couldn't I go? I thought; I'll be quiet—you won't even know I'm in there! Nope, that won't work, he said. In fact, he started just getting up and leaving whenever I would leave the room. I would fix dinner; we would eat; then, while I was in the kitchen cleaning up, he would silently pick up and go! It was unnerving. It was like he would vanish into thin air! When I tried to call him on his cell phone, he wouldn't answer. I would jump in my car and drive all around, trying to find him. Then I would talk myself into going back home again. What are you doing? I would say to myself. Just go home and go to sleep; he'll come home eventually. I would pray and tell God to please protect his crazy son and bring him home safely. "I can't help him, you have to!" I would say.

I couldn't stop him from leaving, and I never knew when he would come home. I couldn't sleep very well, and I would be so angry that I would just lie there, fuming. Sometimes, I would write a two or three page letter to him about how ridiculous he was acting. "Selfish, self-centered, childish" were some of the ways I described this aggravating behavior. I had no way of knowing that this whole thing was going to get much worse or that he couldn't help it. Anyway, I could never give him the letters. He wasn't in the mood to take suggestions or criticism. I knew that if I really blew up and told him how I felt, he wouldn't be able to take it.

I hated to see him like this, and I just couldn't ignore it. I could never count on him to be where he said he would be, and it just got worse. He kept saying stuff like, "You just want to control me!" I thought about that a lot. Yes, I would have liked to control some things, but I knew that we used to have a good relationship. That wasn't just a dream I had. We really did. We had always called each other and let the other one know what was happening. We always told each other goodbye and gave a kiss before parting. Yes, it was your standard, two people in love relationship, but not now.

For a few months it went on like this until one day, I just couldn't hold it in anymore. I have never been able to hold stuff in and act like everything is okay, when it isn't. In fact, I have always, pretty much, told too much of what I thought. You don't actually have to say everything that is on your mind. You should weigh it all out and then thoughtfully say stuff in a positive manner. Yeah, that's the ideal, not always the reality. Well, on this day I just lost it. I yelled—I mean I really yelled. I felt like my husband had been stolen, and I was living with some alien jerk from another planet! So, I told him that. I just didn't know if I could continue with this torturous behavior on his part.

"Someday, I will have had enough of this," I warned, "and then, it will just be over between us!" I was really scared. That's why I said all that, because I had already been divorced before, twenty years earlier. I didn't want to go through that again.

Okay, I'm just going to tell you what I thought at this point, and later I'm going to tell you what God showed me about myself and my marriage that I didn't even know. This just proves that God knows us better than we know ourselves. I thought about what an impossible situation it would be to get a divorce at this point in my life. Hey, I'm not as adventurous, young, or patient as I was back then. I just didn't want the hassle and paperwork of it all! Does that sound cold? Well there you go. That's how I thought it was. I thought that I would soon reach the end of my emotional rope, all traces of whatever love I had for him would be snuffed out, and yes, I would have to sort through my furniture and give him some. No, I didn't want that—not that! My furniture and stuff isn't all that great, but it is mine. All this yelling was also accompanied by a lot of crying (really uncontrollable crying) and stomping around.

As you can guess, that didn't go over too well. I wasn't trying to be theatrical; it just came out really big because I had been holding it in for so long. He didn't like it at all. He got really angry. Then he started telling me that I had threatened divorce and given him an ultimatum. Get over this or else! was what he heard. I didn't mean it that way. I just wanted him to see how his actions were affecting our relationship, and I was being honest when I said that I didn't think I could take it much longer. I truly thought that he would think about what I said and later, come to his senses about it all.

This conversation began a several month period where my husband lived in the same house with me, but tried to avoid seeing me and interacting with me on a daily basis. He acted as if I had done some terrible thing to him; and he now had to consider whether he could stand to be around me anymore at all (that's what he said). Every day, I thought he would snap out of it, but he never did.

Finally, a member at our church who had gone through severe depression took me aside at church one day and told me that I needed to get help for Dave. She had seen the warning signs because she had suffered with severe depression herself. She said that he might not make it if I didn't. I hadn't ever thought about it like that before. I didn't know anything about this kind of depression. I didn't realize that Dave was stricken with a horrible, lonely sadness and became angry at me because he thought I was the one who caused it. He had not seen a doctor about it and just kept thinking that circumstances around him were driving him to feel the way he did. I guess it's normal to blame your spouse when you don't know what's wrong with you.

I did feel bad about this. I tried with all my might to be the nicest, most wonderful wife you can imagine. I thought about every word before I spoke. I prayed constantly for him (not a bad idea anyway—I still do this), but try as I might, he still acted as if he couldn't stand me anymore. Okay, I'm still the same woman (pretty much) he married, so what happened? I felt that God was trying to open my eyes about Dave's problem. I began praying earnestly about talking to him. I prayed for a week before I found a time when I thought I could bring it up. I had a hard time getting it out of my mouth. I was afraid he would be angry at me for thinking he needed a professional, but I had no choice if I wanted to get help for him. I calmly explained the situation and told him that I was not sure how long our relationship could take the strain. He knew we were on shaky ground, and he didn't want to break up; so he agreed, not wholeheartedly, but he agreed anyway.

I prayed again for God to help me find the right doctor or counselor (a Christian). I searched the internet listings and found several nearby. I prayed again for several days and then I called. I made the appointment, and he went. I felt like we were finally getting somewhere.

By this time, God and I were on very close terms. Every other thought was a plea for His help. Dave was so touchy. I counted the days until the newly prescribed depression meds would start helping. They just made him feel groggy, and he didn't like that. He would have to have counseling to help him deal with all the feelings he was having and continue to try to find meds that would work. Rats—this was not coming along very well! I had no idea the process would be so long and drawn out. The doctors told Dave it would take a long time and that he definitely needed a vacation. They told him that his anxiety level was dangerously high and they thought he might have a heart attack or a stroke. The pressure of school, the church, and our relationship was too much. Something had to go. Every time Dave got anxious about something he would say, "You're killing me!"; and he meant it, literally. It was not the church, not the school job, but me who was killing him.

How could that be? I began to feel more and more grieved over this. I was trying to help him (as always), not hurt him. I loved him even though he was perhaps, at that time, one of the most obnoxious humans on the planet. I read as much as I could about depression, anxiety, and ADD on the internet. These are all the things the doctors diagnosed him with. It wasn't good. Some people told stories that were very, very discouraging. I knew that it would be some time before he got better because he was really "bad off."

Our church family tried to be supportive, but it was hard for them. Some people there had some experience with depression, but this wasn't like their depression. It was a lot more severe, and all this anger and resentment just didn't make sense to them. We know now that after the initial physical sickness set in, a spiritual and emotional battle also settled over Dave. He was down and the enemy knew it. It was time to pull out all the stops! It was party time for Satan. With Dave's thinking clouded, all kinds of bad choices would follow.

I knew Satan had gotten involved—somehow I could feel it. Dave wasn't himself, and it was like he was doing everything he could to drive me away and make me hate him for it. I prayed for God to reveal this to Dave. I renounced the enemy. I did this a lot. When Dave was around, I would pray silently for God to defeat whatever demon was whispering in his ear. I had never been taught about spiritual oppression. I knew that Dave was not possessed, but he was being influenced in a completely negative way to act like he had never acted before. He was very cold to me at this time, and I was chilled sometimes when he was around. I went all over our house and dabbed anointing oil on the doors and on his favorite easy chair! Keep away, you ugly devil! I would pray. I was not talking about my husband, but about the presence that seemed to just "arrive" with him most of the time. My stomach would turn over, and every nerve in my body would be tingling. I had no power to remove this invisible foe. I tried, though. I kept thinking that if I kept up the praying, the thing, whatever it was, would not get its way.

You might think all of this is crazy or fanatical, but it's not! I felt an evil presence at this time, and I had not married a person who was like that. For sixteen years I had lived a fairly normal life and had been happy, as well. This guy was different. There was no smiling and laughing, only negative comments, only negative ideas. He was the opposite of the kind and caring man that used to be my husband.

Chapter 20

At the beginning of the summer of 2008, Dave and his doctor decided that he was going on a trip—alone. The doctor told him that if he could get away by himself for awhile, it might help alleviate some of the stress that had built up and take some pressure off. He said he needed to sort things out. He needed to have time to think and relax undisturbed. Dave didn't know for sure where he was going; he was just going to go away by himself. Okay, but we have never taken any vacations away from each other. Dave said that this was not a vacation. He was deeply disturbed and kept thinking that he could get some relief from his awful depression by thinking through everything that was happening.

In theory, I guess, things can be "thought out" and solved. That's if you can think logically. But when your feelings are turned upside down through a chemical imbalance and you are angry with God (rebellion) and angry at those close to you, who you think are making it worse, how can further solitude help? Dave tells about this in his depression story. My own challenge while he was away was to come face-to-face with my own fears.

I asked him to call me from time to time on his trip; and he said, "Okay, but don't call me, I'll call you." "I took that to mean that he really didn't want to be bothered with me unless he felt like it. Why can't I talk to my own husband?" I thought. I felt so alone, abandoned, and unwanted. I knew then that he didn't care about my feelings anymore. That hurt. He had already told me before this, many times, that he just didn't feel anything, that he just didn't care. He wished he did, but he didn't.

Even though Dave was acting like this, I knew that God loved me. I didn't feel loved. I felt ugly, old, wrinkled up, and worthless. But I knew better. I know that who I am to God is not based on how I feel about myself or how others feel about me. To God, I'm the cream-of-the-crop! I'm his masterpiece and his precious child (so are you!). He loves me more than I can ever imagine. This is one area that I have always been positive about. I knew that I had to get very close to my Lord because I needed a hug—not just a hug for then, but an arm around my shoulder for however long this ordeal was going to last. I didn't know how long I could take this rejection from my husband. I thought that at some point I would probably have to stop hoping and face the reality that he was just gone from me (more in spirit than anything else).

How long would I be able to hold myself together? I had to function in the world, take care of my home and myself. It might be weeks, months, or even longer. I just didn't know.

I had been so preoccupied with praying for David that I had not thought about my own well-being. I hadn't been able to sleep or eat properly for six months. I had trouble concentrating on anything except trying to be there for my husband. My heart was broken. I was wounded and hurting, and I was the well one! I turned to my God. What do people do in these circumstances when they don't have a faith in something other than themselves?

I spent a lot of time with my Bible. I began reading in Psalms. King David had faced so many awful times in his life when Saul was hunting him down with armies of thousands to kill him. I felt that this situation was similar. I had a strong inner voice that kept telling me this ordeal was more complicated than it looked. I knew that Dave had been diagnosed with mental illness, but I also knew in my spirit that he was being chased and oppressed by an evil presence.

I refused to let that ugly thing get to me. I was very afraid for my husband's safety, my marriage, and myself. So, I called out to God by claiming all those promises that King David claimed in the scriptures. I prayed over each one, and then I wrote in a journal about how it applied to me. I rewrote those Psalms one at a time, with my name and my situation in them. I knew that the God who protected the hunted David of the Bible was my daddy who was going to protect me.

That was the first fear that hung over me. What will happen to me? My husband has abandoned me. He said he was coming back, but would he? I cowered in my bed with my Bible next to me. I clung to that book, literally. The Lord would show me in the months to come that this fear did not come from Him. The more I read my Bible, prayed, and claimed its truth, the more the fear would subside. I did this every night until I could get calm enough to sleep.

I realized that I had not trusted God as much as this ever before. I had put my trust in my husband to protect me (That is a part of his job.), but I was not totally dependent on God. I was dependent on my husband, who he was, and how he treated me. God gently pried my white-knuckled fingers off of this idea.

Every person we love will let us down at some point (Hopefully, not to this extent!), but our Lord God will never leave us alone. He was in the process of proving to me that He alone deserves my total worship and devotion. My love for my husband did not diminish as I thought it might. God began to change the way I thought about Him, Dave, myself, and what love really is.

Love is the way God treats us. Everything He does is tempered by it. The way we love is nothing like God's love. It's not in us to automatically love like He does. He has to change us in order for that to happen. I had to change the way I thought so that I could survive, mentally. I had to give up my desire to be angry at Dave. That wasn't easy.

I had to give up the temptation to be resentful, as well. That didn't happen overnight. But I knew that's what God wanted me to do. How did I know it? He told me. The only way I could fight this awful thing was to not fight. I tried that to begin with, and it made matters worse. There is no defense against Love. Love can move mountains, and Love can heal any hurt. God is Love. So, God had to do it all. Basically, I realized I was incapable of doing anything that would help.

Here is the scripture that describes God's love in the Bible: "Love is patient. Love is kind. It does not envy. It does not boast. It is not proud. It is not rude. It is not self-seeking. It is not easily angered. It keeps no record of wrongs."

(1 Corinthians 13:4-5) Several years ago, I put this scripture on my refrigerator, and the Holy Spirit began to tell me that this was very important for me. He told me this long before I knew what He was talking about.

Throughout David's depression, I would look at this scripture on my fridge, and I would think, Well, my husband is the very opposite of this right now. He was not patient and never kind anymore. He was rude, seeking to help himself, not me. He got angry all the time and remembered every wrong ever done to him and some that I thought he just imagined. He took things I said in the wrong way most of the time, and he was generally impossible to live with.

God kept telling me that I had to be more like this scripture. Patience had to be unending. You can't blow up at a sick person. It makes them feel worse, and I surely did not want to make Dave feel worse! Every time I woke in the night, burdened for him, I wanted to say, Hey buddy, you brought this on yourself, somehow. You've pushed me away, and so you don't deserve to get any more help from me. However, the Holy Spirit would correct me every time, and I would pray instead for David's protection.

I wanted to get comfort from my husband; I needed him to be kind or affectionate, even slightly, but he just wouldn't. But "Love is not self-seeking." God was telling me that what I wanted wasn't going to happen right now, so not to dwell on it.

I had so much trouble with anger. I couldn't let it out on Dave, so I would hold it in and think all kinds of bad things about him. I called him names and accused him of every bad thing that I could think of in my mind. I knew this had to go. I have had the habit throughout our marriage of thinking certain ugly things about him whenever I was mad. Namely, I thought he was an idiot and a big jerk. This habit was just enlarged, and I felt totally justified, at first. Then that line, "Love is not easily angered," came to mind. I asked God to forgive me for thinking like that. He had to help me a lot because this was hard. I didn't realize that it was such a sin until God revealed it to me. It affected me. It made me feel worse than ever to be so angry at him.

The last area the verse talks about is this: "Love keeps no record of wrongs." This was the hardest one for me. I like to keep up with what someone has done against me. That way, I can tell them about it. I can also keep up with any pattern that is forming.

I mean, I needed to be able to mentally link all those bad deeds against me together and form a picture of what was going on, right? Wrong! There's no way we can live in peace and hold resentments against others, especially those we love. That's not godlike love. That meant, therefore, that every time Dave did another rude or uncaring thing, I had to forgive him right there and not carry it over to the next day. I had to forget it! That was not easy for me, either. Resentment over the way I was being unjustly treated was the hardest temptation for me.

I had done nothing to deserve this mental abuse, but that isn't mentioned in the scripture. It doesn't say, Love keeps no record of wrongs except when you don't deserve it! You see, this stuff is not human. We want to be angry and resentful at those who spitefully use us; it's only natural, but the Bible says love them instead. You don't ever think that the spiteful stuff will come from your best friend. I desperately wanted to learn how to do this. Only God's Holy Spirit puts this kind of desire in us. The want to be more like Him was what got me through the hardest times. To be totally free of resentment and anger is a freedom like no other. The pain of all that stuffed down in your spirit is a prison, and it hurts you more than you know. It eventually hurts our relationship with God, and most of the time we don't even realize it.

I constantly reminded myself of what Jesus Christ endured for me. He went through so much more than we can imagine, and He did it all for love! He reminded me that I have done wrong things and thought in rebellious ways, at times, as well. The Bible teaches that all sin is reprehensible to God. My sin was condemning for me, yet He forgave me.

The scripture teaches that we must forgive others. Mathew chapter 6 says: "If you don't forgive others your heavenly father will not forgive you." It's not an option.

I respect my heavenly Father. I needed His help. I wanted to be obedient and submissive to what He expected of me. I told Him that I was His girl from now on. Whatever He wanted me to do, I would do it. I meant it. My soul cried out to Him. There was always just enough peace for that day; the next day I would have to earnestly ask Him for more.

My chest would ache over all this. Even though I had faith in God, the temptation to break down was always there. I was honest with Him about it all. He heard my frustration and fears daily. I cried a lot. Some days were worse than others, but there always seemed to be one little bright spot that would lift me up.

My family called frequently and friends would also. I got cards from time to time, and I knew people were praying. I can't tell you how much I appreciated the support of others. Every time someone called or came over, I thanked God for sending them. He always knew when I really needed a live person to encourage me. It's funny, I had always been the one to call or encourage other people. Now, I was the needy one; and I realized that I was vulnerable (not a good feeling for me) to all the attacks of fear and loneliness that the enemy was hurling my way. I didn't feel strong or courageous at all. I felt weak, and I didn't understand until much later what God was going to do.

Chapter 21

Dave finally called me and said he was on his way home. He told me about all the places he had visited in order to reconnect with who he really was. It sounds funny to think that you can lose yourself, doesn't it? It didn't help for me to tell him who he was. He actually remembered being different, but he didn't feel like the Godly person he used to be. He just felt like a loser, a failure, and totally worthless. Remember that the devil is a liar. That's all he knows how to do. He can't tell the truth. Even though it didn't help (at that time), I kept telling him this.

While he was driving, he kept telling me that he had missed me and that our love would heal him. Well, that sounds kind of mushy and nice to hear, but it gave me an uneasy feeling. If our love could heal him, how come it hadn't done it already? I knew that this was not the answer, but I wanted him to come home. He had told me about the drinking and sleeping in his car all the time. I had given him up to God in this area, but I hated to think that was how he was living.

He told me he had visited a family we knew and his own family while he was gone, and I thought that was a good thing. I think the most important thing about it was that even though he had been totally alone most of the time and did a whole lot of thinking, it hadn't changed the fact that he was still depressed and chemically unbalanced. Running away didn't fix anything! It just made him see that he still felt rotten with or without me around. He said that he realized it wasn't me that was causing this whole thing. That was a relief!

I wanted him to try a different medication that I had seen on TV and the internet. He asked his doctor about it and got some to try. I was hoping this would get his emotions balanced out. He still had anxiety attacks and severe mood swings daily. I trusted God for the answers, but I know that sometimes God uses doctors, medicines, counselors, and other things to bring healing.

I knew that it all had to happen in God's timeframe, but I couldn't figure out what was taking Him so long. When things are going great, time just flies; but when you or a loved one is in misery, time drags on and on.

Over the next few months, Dave would feel better, try to come back to himself, then feel worse and go downhill again. The meds would work for a while and then," boom," he would hit rock bottom again. It was a roller coaster of emotions for us both and the most difficult thing that either one of us has ever experienced.

As I have said before, healing came in the Lord's time and neither one of us knew when it would happen or even if it would. I believed that God's plan for me would include healing no matter what happened to Dave and at times I thought almost anything could happen!

When Dave was at his worst, I could actually feel a pressure that was almost unbearable. My body hurt, I had to force myself to eat, and I had a terrible time sleeping at night. I know that there was a great deal of spiritual warfare going on. The only thing I could do was claim the promises of God from His word and pray for healing and protection for Dave. By this time, I had forgotten how to smile most of the time. Smiling has been my habit most of my life (I come from a jolly family of "smilers"); but now, I couldn't think of anything to smile about. I was sad, very sad, and tired of suffering emotionally with no end in sight.

I was just waiting on God—and it wasn't easy to do! I admire people who say they go through things and the peace of God just keeps them safe. I was safe, but all this turmoil had taken a toll on my own self-worth and well-being. I didn't know how much until God sent a very specific word of encouragement to me through some people from Central Assembly who are gifted in the prophetic ministry.

If you look in 1 Corinthians Chapter 12, verses 1-12, you will see the spiritual gifts listed. The scripture says that all these gifts are given for the common good of the body. As Christians we are the body of Christ that is mentioned here. I have never been to a church before where the gift of prophecy has been used to encourage people, but this was a wonderful experience! I was not expecting to get a message from the Lord, but that is exactly what happened. These kind people did not know who I was or what I was going through. They just prayed for me, and God revealed to them some things that He wanted me to know. I didn't realize that Dave's depression was affecting me so profoundly, but of course, God knows at all times what we are going through and is intensely aware of our sufferings.

It was near the end of January 2009, and I had a strong desire to attend a church in Vero Beach that Dave had visited several years before. He had been uplifted there; and every time we passed by their building, on our way to a movie or to the mall (in the years before his depression), we would comment, "Someday we are going to visit there." I believe God had placed in us the desire to go there long before we ever knew that we had a need for the restoration that would come from that very place!

I was so sad and down that day. It was a Sunday morning, and some friends had said they would like to come with me. Some men in the lobby greeted us warmly, and one in particular told me that I should check out the prophetic ministry after the service. Not knowing what this consisted of, but open to anything positive, I said I would. I thought maybe there was a group of people who would pray with you about your problems; and I wanted to pray for my husband.

After the service I went over to the designated area and waited. I tried hard not to think of anything, because it was a struggle at this point not to cry constantly. I didn't really want to open up about my problems and let it all out. I had been holding things in for so long; it had become my way of life.

Soon I was in a small Sunday school room with two kind mannered people. I had gotten an instruction sheet, which told me to just quietly wait and receive a word of encouragement after a few minutes of prayer. The man and woman closed their eyes and began to pray silently. I did the same. I told God that I needed His help and I wanted to hear anything that He had to tell me. All this was a little surprising, because I thought I was going to be praying for Dave. I didn't know that God had planned this for me.

The lady said, "I see a beautiful gate. It is shut and locked. At one time it would open freely, and wonderful things would flow in and out of the gate from heaven to earth and from earth back to heaven. But now it is closed tight. Something happened a year or so ago that caused it to be closed and locked."

I knew right away that the gate was my heart and the wonderful things were ministries and words to others that I was used to saying and doing because of my joy in the Lord. When my husband began to reject me and then continued on his self-destructive path, I was so concentrated on him and our problems that I no longer saw opportunities of ministry around me. I had become closed and protective of my space. I have always been unafraid to be myself; but now, I didn't think I had anything left to share with anyone. I didn't realize how side-tracked I had become! I have always loved being friendly and doing things for others, but that was not happening at all anymore.

The young man said, "God wants you to know that He loves how soft and easy you are to others. You readily speak to anyone and are very comfortable with people you don't even know. He loves this about you." Wow! This made me feel so warm inside. There was no way these people could have guessed all this stuff. I always have felt comfortable being friendly with just about anyone and am always looking for ways to help someone or lift them up. Sometimes, I have to tell myself to stop it! You're getting ridiculous; you don't even know these people. (My kids have said this.)

Then the lady said, "You are getting burned. It's like you are walking on hot coals all the time. God is holding you up to keep you from getting burned, but you are absorbing the fire anyway." Even though, by now, I knew Dave wasn't himself, many times his actions and words hurt me deeply. That was the burning she was referring to! I knew God was sending people to give the words I needed, and my Bible held many words of encouragement as well. No matter how much I tried, though, I couldn't get my mind off my husband and how much he desperately needed help.

However, all these statements were meaningful to me. I recognized that they had to come from God. No person can read your mind or look at you and come up with a spiritual analogy that describes what you are or have been going through. It made me so happy to know that God wanted to tell me these things. It was just as if He spoke them to me Himself, and I was tremendously cheered by this!

Then the lady said, "We are going to pray for you now, for healing." She put her hands on my head and prayed for the wounded areas in my mind and the burnt areas that had been damaged. I felt a cool sensation, like a gentle flowing of water in my head. I felt peacefulness and calm settle over me like a mist from a waterfall that I had somehow been sitting near. I felt a new awareness that God wanted me to be myself again. Somehow, I had lost the real me, just as my husband had. I just needed someone to tell me, because I didn't have a chemical imbalance to battle through.

After this, I had a renewed hope. I had been refreshed by God's presence in a way I had never experienced before. This was just the beginning of my learning more about how our Savior planned to send healing, not only to Dave, but to me, also. Hallelujah! I will never be the same!

Chapter 22

By this time, Dave was not living at home anymore. He had been staying at his mother's house. It was empty, and he didn't have the patience to deal with any relationships. Every week, he would struggle to get through his work at school; and then when Friday afternoon came around, he would be gone. He would hop in his car, drive to somewhere, drink, sleep in parking lots, or walk around alone. He was in too much pain to face the people he loved, but he would spend time talking to total strangers—at car shows or flea markets—about meaningless stuff. He would come back Sunday night because he had to be at work the next day.

Where in the heck was he going? What in the world was he doing when he got there? Whom was he talking to, and what in God's name were they talking about? All these questions were constantly running through my mind like a freight train. I don't like it when I don't know what is going on. Maybe you're like that too. I had always trusted my husband; but now, it was a whole different story.

I had a difficult time concentrating on God instead of this lunatic that somehow had invaded my husband's body. But I kept hearing God's voice in my head say, Don't pay any attention to what he does and especially ignore most of what he says! If that didn't go against my grain, nothing would. If anything, my habit in life is to pay really close attention; otherwise, somebody might sneak up and steal something from you. Is this starting to sound like I have a problem with trust that I didn't know I had?

It was not that challenging to trust a husband who obviously adores and cares intensely for you; but when the circumstances changed dramatically, I struggled. For one thing, Dave had taken off his wedding ring about five months earlier and put it somewhere. (I couldn't find it—I looked!)

This was like a stab in the heart, and every time I saw his naked finger with the white part where the ring used to be, my wounded heart would bleed more. I had to bite my lip to not mention this obviously ugly and rejecting act, but it did no good to talk about it. I recall that I was really angry back then. He had said some angry stuff, huffed around, and bolted straight out the door.

I remember I was feeling my usual "I-could-slap-the-next-person-who-moves" emotion after he left, and I could do nothing about it. I got in the shower and began telling God what a low down, unbelievable fool I was married to. I began to think, Okay, what if I take my ring off until he puts his back on? I easily slipped my ring off my wet finger and immediately heard in my head a very firm, Put that back on! You are not going to act like that. You are not going to play games. I hurriedly put my ring on because I knew it was the wrong thing to do.

God expected me to keep on repaying all this evil with good. No matter how awful and negative our relationship was going to get, the Lord wanted me to hang in there and be supportive, loving, kind, and yes, even forgiving. I didn't know it at the time, but God had planned to give me just as much faith and endurance as I asked Him for. He had also planned to send people to help me when I needed help. I didn't know He was going to be so faithful and good to me. I didn't know that the bond that had been placed between me and my husband was supernaturally reinforced by God himself. I was just too afraid.

From that day when Dave took his ring off and left to live away from me, the spiritual attacks got worse. The pressure of them was something that never left me. I knew that our home and our friendship were being tested in a way I never thought was possible. I tell you the truth—it was not in me to hang in there; it was God's idea. He was the one who told me what He wanted me to do, and it was the opposite of what I felt like doing! It's all laid out in that scripture that tells what real love is. And as I said before, this kind can only come from God.

So by the time I got to the point of receiving this word of encouragement from these God-sent people at Central

Assembly, I was pretty beat up emotionally and spiritually from the battle in my own heart to be there for Dave, while questioning it all at the same time. I kept asking myself, How much of this is the chemical imbalance, and how much is pure out-and-out sin?

God let me know that He was in charge of that category. He could handle it; I couldn't. I couldn't figure it out either. I had to trust Him even if I couldn't trust my husband any-more. Believe me; I was tired after a year and a half of tur-moil like this. As the months had passed, it was no easier to handle. It had become a lot more difficult; and this word from God changed everything about how I felt.

I think God was taking me off the case—my husband's case—and putting me back in charge of my own case. I have found out a lot of things about spiritual authority since then. God had not released me from the bond of friendship and marriage no matter what the other person had done or said, but He wanted me to concentrate on my own walk with Him and leave everything else to Him. I still felt the mounting pressure, but I knew He was in control.

Two weeks after I got this encouraging word from the pro-phetic team at Central, Dave actually showed up at church, proclaimed he was healed, and came home for good. Healing can be just around the corner, and we don't even know it. I think that the enemy put in his last big push to drive Dave and me over the edge right before the battle was won. I don't know how to tell you the way it was to make you understand, but it was a real miracle. Something in the world around me was changed. Something had been defeated. Someone had won a war. I was a bystander, a participant, a victim, an ad-vocate, and a beat-up winner, all at once!

You may think, How could you tell it was real? That was my first thought, as well! I was relieved and grateful to the Lord. I wanted to trust that God had done what friendship, time, and medicine could not. I had told Him that I would forgive my husband and put all the hurt in the past. My heart was right in this area, but my mind kept nagging at me with questions and reminders of all too many wounds that were still fresh. I didn't know that it would take a face-to-face encounter with God (for both Dave and me) to get this part of our healing accomplished.

Chapter 23

When Dave and I met the pastor and his wife, they immediately took us under their wing. Again, I say this was God's whole idea! He knew where we needed to be, and somehow He got us there! We were going to a church in a town fifty-four miles away for a reason. God always does things for a reason.

They prayed with us, encouraged us both, and promised to be there for us as we recovered. This pastor was moved to work with my husband right from the beginning. He put his arm around him and told him that he believed in him. He cried with him over the pain he had experienced. That meant everything to Dave. I think it was because he knew that he didn't deserve to be treated so well. He had made mistakes and didn't feel worthy to be welcomed like this. He had been far away from God for a while and fighting to get back at the same time.

I want to describe to you what he looked like at this point because I think it makes a big difference in how you picture this process. He was a mess. Because he had stopped caring about himself, he had gained some weight. Because he went most of the time on three or four hours of sleep, he was bleary eyed and puffy. He was clean, but wore an old, black biker T-shirt, worn-out jeans, and sandals. His hair was the worst! It was down to his shoulders, raggedy, and unkempt. My former handsome, neat, and tidy husband looked like a homeless, old woman dressed up like an old biker! I loved him anyway because he was alive and in one piece, but I was concerned about what the rest of the world would think about him. But, honestly, you couldn't tell that anyone at this church noticed at all.

The pastor greeted him warmly with a hug and was so kind to this guy who looked like a vagabond. I was kind of thin, having lost weight from not eating, and red-eyed by then, as well. I had no makeup on for the first month we attended there because as soon as the praise and worship would start, all the tears I cried (from relief) would wash it all off! Yes, I was also a sorry sight. But we were treated kindly by everyone and especially that pastor and his wife. The funny thing is that they were dressed very nicely, so you would think they would not want to be seen with a bum-looking guy and his skinny, runny-nosed wife. But, that was the opposite of the way they acted.

We went to every service—three times a week, and this pastor sought us out after every service to take us out to eat and talk. We felt as if we were special because of this treatment, and we didn't even know why they would take so much time with people who lived out of town, weren't members of their church and obviously had issues. They acted as if they really enjoyed our company and wanted to be with us. It made us feel like real people again. How could nicely dressed, successful, and happy church people want to hang out with such obvious losers? That is really how we felt, and we were so grateful for all the positive attention from them. I never heard one critical word from them, only encouragement and lots of smiles.

This guy was funny! It was just what the doctor (Doctor Jesus) had ordered. We laughed constantly at all his jokes, and he was so jovial about everything! He lifted that feeling of dread about what we had been through, whenever we were around him. He is a warm, kind, and sensitive man, who is a "barrel of fun" all at the same time.

One evening, after a Sunday night service, we were talking over dinner when the pastor's wife invited me to go to a ladies' encounter. I had been to lots of retreats and ladies get-togethers as a pastor's wife before, so I thought this was probably the same type of uplifting event.

She explained that it was a two day weekend with other women from the church. I eagerly accepted because I knew that I needed uplifting and time to process all that had happened to us. It was scheduled for about two and a half weeks from then, about five weeks after we started going to church there and since Dave's healing. Since they only did these encounters a few times per year, I felt fortunate that the timing allowed for me to make it to one so soon. I had no earthly idea what I was going to be experiencing. I just trusted this nice lady who seemed to think that this was just what I needed!

I didn't know that she saw more than just my skinny self and worn-out face. She saw a need for spiritual renewing and healing. She saw a need for real instruction and encouragement in forgiveness (God wanted to make sure I really learned this). I would have to say that the Lord told her all this, because she just knew it. I still struggled with the crying bit, not knowing why; but this restoring and renewing business is something that this pastor, his wife, and church are well acquainted with. This is their business, and they are very serious about getting it done! As I found out at the encounter, spiritual healing may not be easy, but it is needed. I couldn't move on from where I was until I got it. It's not a crime to be wounded and worn. It's not unreasonable at all. But you don't want to stay that way.

Jesus died for more than that. It says in the scriptures, "By His stripes we are healed!" It doesn't say, some of you or someday. It says "we are." The problem is that there has to be a mental lifting of burdens to feel our healing. The pain from wounds that have been inflicted upon us and wounds we have caused others can linger forever if we don't get free of it.

I guess you're thinking that freedom from pain and freedom from guilt, suffering, and shame are unrealistic. Do I really mean that those heavy weights on my heart can leave and not be in there anymore? Yes, Yes, Yes—Do you see me jumping up right now with joy about this? The encounter was exactly what it's called, an encounter with God!

Chapter 24

Why do we think that our life just happens sometimes? If we pay close attention, we will start to notice that everything, and I mean everything, is happening for a purpose. That purpose could be to bring us closer to God, to bring us through a problem, or to bring us into contact with others where we can help them do the same thing!

It so happened, though I don't think it was a coincidence, that I got a ride to the encounter with two lovely people who blessed me as we traveled. One of them also just happened to be my roommate. God had planned all the details to bring me comfort and encouragement on the way. There were also understanding counselors for every person and wonderful food for every meal, which was home cooked by the staff at the church who hosted the get-together. There was a wing attached to the church where we occupied comfortable, hotel-like rooms.

I didn't know a soul there, though I was fairly familiar with the very nice wife of the pastor. I arrived tired, burdened with my hurt feelings, and a little nervous about these strangers who would be sharing my weekend. I was prepared to look at Bible verses and pray. I figured it would be pretty nice and restful. I didn't know that it would be nothing like that at all.

I can't tell every step of the process because this weekend spiritual renewal depends on the participant's having no preconceived notions about what will occur. I don't want to divulge it all because you may be able to attend something like this one day. I will simply tell you the things I learned about healing and getting closer to God through this deeply moving time of regeneration.

First, and most importantly: I have never truly understood everything I needed to know about the power of God. I thought I did. I thought that on the scale of one to ten in the "know-it-all-about-God range, I was probably a nine. I have been saved since I was twelve, more than forty years; I have been in a church most of the time since then, taught classes, organized all sorts of learning-about-Jesus stuff, and served as a valued advisor to my pastor-husband. I enthusiastically attended all the Sunday school sessions, Bible study classes, and spiritual workshops that came my way. I felt empowered, triumphant, and full of good-will right up till the time my world was jerked into the "twilight zone" for a full eighteen months!

Now I had to come face to face with the fact that I couldn't get myself together in the aftermath of it all. I really thought it might take years to get rid of the knot in my stomach and the continual flow of tears.

The organizers of this weekend kept telling us that this was not a time for us to help one another. It was a time to concentrate on hearing from God. We needed to know what He had to say to us individually, and you can't do that if you are focused on other people. So, I prayed that God would tell me what I needed to know. I wanted to be open to anything He wanted to reveal to me, even though I couldn't imagine that I would learn something that I didn't already know (This is not an attractive thing to admit).

The people who served as leaders at this time had already spent weeks praying and asking God for his help with each one of us. They didn't know any specifics about most of us, especially not me, but they didn't need to. They lifted us up in prayer and prepared for the time we would be spending together by fasting as well.

They were telling God that they were serious about wanting deliverance and freedom for these sisters who had come. They sacrificed their weekend with their families in an unselfish effort to bring us into a closer relationship with Jesus Christ—and it worked. God began to show me things that I already knew but in a way that applied to my hurting self. I had always been able to see things for others, but had let my close, intimate relationship with my Savior slide. Because I thought my priority was helping others, including my husband, I had neglected my own conversations with Him about me.

As I contemplated the unbelievable sacrifice Jesus made on the cross, I realized it was over. Jesus' sacrifice was over—He had won over death and dying. That victory guaranteed that I could now and forever count on Him for everything in my own life. He spoke to my heart of hearts and told me that there was not going to be a continuing of pain; this was the end of it.

He said to my spirit that I no longer had to suffer as I had. He confirmed that the battle was over. Of course this was the spiritual battle I had felt, but couldn't understand fully. I realized that there are some things we don't have to understand, just believe.

It was a very intimate time. I can only say, He held me close and took away my fear of the pain. The constant feeling of grief over how I was treated was removed. I know that this was supernatural. The love that flowed from the Cross to my soul was unmistakable. This was where the real battle had been fought—not in my lifetime, but when Jesus showed His love for me so long ago. Now I could feel the power of God bring a sense of peace that is not able to be humanly explained or expressed. I went to bed that night emotionally drained, but I slept better than I can remember in a long time.

Second: There can be evil influences and oppression in our lives or in those of our loved ones. There are things that we do that open the door to all kinds of influences in our spirit. Some of these are involvements with people whom God never intended us to get involved with or activities and habits that do not glorify God. Plainly put, some of this stuff is put in our path by the enemy of all Christians, Satan. The Bible speaks of the problems we can incur just because the Earth is inhabited not only by man; it is also the kingdom and realm of the fallen angel, Lucifer (now called Satan), and a third of the angels of heaven who rebelled with him. These fallen angels are demons whose job it is to plague man with any and all kinds of unholy things that they can come up with. And they can come up with plenty!

As I have said before, it's not a matter of blaming all bad things on the Devil. It is a matter of realizing that there is a spiritual world inhabited with powerful angels of protection and assistance sent from God as well as those bent on destructiveness and death as directed by Satan. I believe we can see the increased demonic activity in our world today, as more drug, alcohol, sexual perversion, and despicable crimes against human kind seem to be increasing and even accepted by many.

Whether by association of ourselves with the devil or that of our relatives (generational curses and sins), these demonic forces seem to get attached to us and can hang on for a lifetime. Many addictions and diseases seem to run in families and whether a product of the fallen world we live in or the result of demonic oppression, this spiritual force meant for our downfall does not have to be ignored or put up with!

The power of God is far greater in these areas, but we have to recognize the source of the influence and seek the Lord's hand for victory over these destructive enemies! He is with us. So, who can be against us?

We must understand this is not a reason to be fearful, but a reason to know who we are in Christ Jesus; and we are not to think that we have to live under the oppression or influence of Satan. Once one has recognized an unholy presence in his life, for any reason, he should fervently ask God to help him get rid of it! We have the divine right to freedom (when we claim it) through the victory that Jesus won for us. Casting out these fears, doubts, and other barbs thrown at us from hell can be the beginning of real liberation from many things—physical, spiritual, and emotional—that have plagued us for years.

Like God, we are a three-part being: physical, emotional, and spiritual (God is Father, Son, and Holy Spirit). We cannot ignore that there is a spiritual world of good and evil around us. Don't forget though, two thirds of the angels stayed true to God; so that means the good angels outweigh the bad two to one! They also have the Almighty God as their commander and because He has made them and all of us, He holds the master plan for our good!

Third: Forgiveness must be final and lasting for all others in our lives, because that's how He forgives us. Sometimes we don't even know that we have an attitude that creates a wall or a hindrance between ourselves and others. Sometimes we do. Thinking that it is okay to carry unforgiveness against others is a worldly way of thinking and it is proliferated by hell itself.

As long as we have a block in our emotions against someone else, we have a block between us and God. Even if someone has done wrong by us, we do not have the right to be unforgiving.

We think that if we cast them away from us or "move on" with our relationships or friendships it's okay. It is not. Other people in our lives must know that we have forgiven them. That releases them from any guilt or resentment they may feel. It doesn't mean a relationship will be restored or that we must be best friends with everyone. That's not going to happen; however, forgiveness is freedom for the forgiver, first and foremost.

If you think there are some things you cannot forgive, you are right! Some things are just not humanly possible to forgive, even when we want to. That's why God gets involved, prompting us by what he said in the Bible. "Remember to forgive others as you have been forgiven" is a commandment not a suggestion. Persisting in holding up these "walls" of unforgiveness toward others will affect us spiritually, and God will eventually do what He has to do so that we will be restored to Him.

Forgiving is an ongoing thing. It means that whenever a thought that would remind us of past hurts comes up, we recognize it and cast it out! I am not going down that road! is what I think to myself, because I certainly want to be forgiven for my sins as long as I live. I know I will never be without sin, as the Bible reminds us, and so I will always need to foster this habit of forgiving and forgetting.

"I can forgive, but I can't forget," I have heard people say. This sentiment is "hogwash!" You have forgotten many things, like your own mistakes, for example; and God can do anything in you when it is His will. Maybe you won't entirely forget, but at least you can remember the reason why you are not dwelling on it. Ask Him for help with this and don't be so stubborn about it!

I am saying all this to myself as well, because I think the longer we live and the more we rub elbows with other people—the only way to live—the more chance we have of getting hurt. Sometimes, that pain comes from those we love and believe in the most!

Chapter 25

Everyone who went to the weekend encounter was at church that Sunday. When we came into the auditorium, all the women who went, including the leaders, were so happy and so free that you could feel the waves of excitement in the room! Some gave testimonies, and some told of long held hurts and problems that they had received help and healing for. I was filled with a deep sense of awe at what the power of God can do in the lives of people who believe and claim it! I had a wonderful peace and an overwhelming sense of who I was again.

When we become entrenched in a battle for our loved ones, our sanity, and our very lives, we can get battle weary and full of wounded places. That's how I felt going into the encounter with God. But in the following weeks, after these "revelations of truth," which came directly from God's heart to mine that weekend, I walked in a new peace and purpose. I became unburdened of pain that I had held not only during the many months of my husband's depression, but also of many emotional wounds that had occurred in my past.

He opened my eyes to what forgiveness can do for me and those I choose to forgive. He taught me that my marriage was a supernaturally inspired and supported union that could not be easily broken. I saw the work of Satan in our lives as a daily and ongoing assault, which we have the power to resist and even cast out.

The most important thing I learned from this experience is this: I need God because He is mighty and awesome when I am weak and alone. He loves me and He wants me to trust Him more. I have to seek Him to reveal what I feel, but can't explain. One day, when I see Him, I will understand. I know it will be worth it all. I respect His authority in my life to do whatever He wills. I trust Him. I respect my husband's authority under God, and I know God will take care of him as well. I am not afraid.

Thank you, dear Jesus—you are a true friend!

Part 3

WHAT
I HAVE
LEARNED

(Pastor Dave)

Chapter 26

The truth is that there are areas of our lives that are vitally important to our spiritual health, and the enemy would like for us to ignore them. Actually, it's a goal of his to distract us with unimportant things or issues that cloud our thinking. When we do so, even unintentionally, he gains a foothold; then he uses them to pry open the door of one's life and barge in, bringing in pain and more unhealthy things with him. I want to explain each of these areas, how they can get out of balance, and then how the stinking enemy came into my life in a big way and put his stamp of approval on the whole mess! Remember, this scenario or story has been a lifelong project for him. He knows our history, weak points, enemies, hurts, and problems. He has assigned workers (demons) who are on our case and are standing at the ready to be used when the time is right.

God has assigned his angels for protection as well; however, certain conditions can cause a rumble in the spiritual world, and we know this as spiritual warfare. The Bible speaks of this extensively with many examples of people who are hounded and subjected to spiritual attack. The Bible also speaks of God's strength and the armies of angels that attend his followers.

If you are under spiritual attack, it can mean several things. It does not mean, however, that God doesn't love you any more or that He has left or abandoned you. He hasn't put in all the time to make you who you are and given you guidance so far in your life to just throw His hands up and say; "I'm done!" People may do that, but not God. Read Romans 8:38-39. He will go to the ends of the Earth for you—to whatever hell you've fallen into or whatever circumstance. He wants you back, and He wants you healthy!

I would like you to know that in no way do I explain away my circumstances by saying, "The devil made me do it!" No, in fact, the thoughts I have expressed here are meant to give you a more complete picture of how our own weaknesses, physical and spiritual, coupled with the attack of Satan, can completely steal our joy, destroy our relationships—the very fabric of our lives—and even kill us! I believe that was the goal of the enemy in my depression. He saw the opportunity of a lifetime (mine!)—the perfect storm, if you will, and he went for it.

I learned so many things about myself, others, and especially God during and after this trial I went through. One thing I learned was that God wanted to use this experience to show me things about myself, which could only be revealed by going through the fire, and I want to share just a few of those with you.

The first thing I want to share with you is about discouragement. The biggest avenue of attack the devil has used on me over the years has been discouragement. I knew this in part, but God revealed it to me in an even greater way after my healing. I believe He allowed me to go through this and come out on the other side for a couple of reasons. For one thing, He wanted me to learn how to be victorious in this area of my life because He has even greater battles for me to fight in the kingdom of God and many souls for me to win and snatch from the fires of hell for Him in the future. If I am discouraged, I cannot be as effective in the battle—and neither can you!

When I was a boy, I used to be teased constantly by my classmates at school because of my teeth. I had very bad buck teeth. I was made fun of a lot by others. I was very self-conscious of this and in later years tried to smile without opening my mouth. I would often talk to others with one hand over my mouth because I was so embarrassed. In fact, the only way I was able to garner any respect at all and avoid the teasing later in high school was to become a good athlete.

That stopped the teasing at the high school level, but it never stopped the low self-esteem that resulted from years of harassment and embarrassment. Even as an adult I heard little jokes made in "good-hearted" fun, but hurtful all the same! I know what it is like to experience ridicule and scorn at an early age, and those experiences can haunt you for a lifetime unless you come to God and let Him bring healing from those childhood hurts. If we only knew how our words can bring blessing or curses on those around us! If we saw the effect with our spiritual eyes, we would never think of uttering one word against another human being. Words can damage for a lifetime unless God is welcomed in with His healing power! And He does heal!

When I was around eleven or twelve years old, I had an experience that really changed my life. You might call it a God moment. I had come home from school one afternoon extremely upset and discouraged, having been made fun of pretty cruelly that day. In fact, I was so upset that I felt as if I had had enough. I remember that I was crying pretty hard. I didn't want to be around anyone, so I went out to the barn. We lived on a small farm in north central Ohio at the time, so being in the barn was not an unusual thing to be doing. It was what I was going to do that afternoon that was different than the usual chores I was accustomed to. I found a long rope and threw it over one of the rafters and tied it off. Then I sat on the top of one of the animal pens and tied the other end around my neck. I tied it so that when I slipped off of the top board on the pen, there would be plenty of space between the barn floor and my feet. I was going to kill myself.

As I sat there and reflected on all the insults and taunting that had occurred, not only that day, but for several school years even before that, I began to cry even harder. You see, the old saying, "sticks and stones can break my bones, but words will never hurt me" is just not true! Words have the power to destroy and curse, or they have the power to bring joy and impart blessing. Kids can be especially cruel to each other, as many of you know. That day the words brought such a sense of discouragement that I didn't want to endure it any longer.

Just as I was ready to slip off of that top board and plunge into eternity, something happened—a voice in my spirit spoke to me just as clearly as if someone present had spoken the words. This voice asked me a simple question, Why do you want to kill yourself? And I actually answered audibly, "People make fun of me all the time because of my teeth, and I don't want to be made fun of anymore!" Then the voice said something to me that dried my tears immediately and made me stop: One day you will be a grown man, and when you are, you will be able to get braces. Then you will never be made fun of again for your teeth. When you are a man, you can then become whatever you want.

I was not a Christian at that time. I had heard the Gospel over and over again, but I resisted the wooing of the Holy Spirit to yield my life to Him. In that moment, however, every tear dried up. Something came over me that gave me a sense of purpose and resolve. I slipped the rope off of my neck, untied it from the rafter and put it back where I had found it. I walked out of the barn knowing I had heard directly from God Himself. The "word" spoken to me that day came to pass years later—at twenty-seven years of age I had braces put on. Three and a half years later they came off. I finally had straight white teeth!

Discouragement is one of the key ways the enemy of our souls has come to steal, kill, and destroy the wonderful things God has planned for us. God wants to encourage us. I have had many discouraging moments over the years, but God wants you and me to learn to be victorious in this area of our lives. How can we do this? I have several thoughts about it.

First, we have to cultivate a close relationship with God through His Son, Jesus Christ. You have to be in a right relationship with Him to the point where He has become your best friend. The Bible says that we are the Bride of Christ, but many people just want to, so to speak, date Him, not marry Him. You and I have to want Him more than we want all the temporary things this world has to offer. Do you remember what it was like when you fell in love? Remember how you couldn't wait to get a letter or phone call from your new "heart-throb"!? Remember how you could spend hours talking on the phone or wondering where the time went after spending an evening together on a date? This is the same way with our Lord. We have to cultivate a relationship where we fall in love with Him—some of us for the first time and some of us all over again!

How do you do this? Spend time getting to know Him. Your relationship with God should be one of closeness and honesty. You can't fool around with God as if He doesn't know that you've got some areas where you don't let Him in. Of course He knows! You can't be flirting around with anything that He has told you is wrong according to the scriptures or anything that He has told you in your heart is wrong for you. Just because others get away with that second glance at a woman or looking at risqué pictures, these actions are not for you! He has set you aside as His. Don't flirt or play with any of these things. You will suffer in your relationship with Him and lose the intimacy that leads to "perfect peace."

Your mind is like a house with many rooms inside. Every area of your life has a room, and every room should be clean. Those dirty rooms can have locked doors where you don't allow anyone in; but God made you, and He knows already what is in every room. You can pretend your house is pristine and clean; and you might even have others around you fooled, but God knows the truth. He will let you know in your spirit that something needs to be done. But if you continually ignore His voice, your own reasoning will come into play.

Your own reasoning always serves the flesh. It is self-serving and focused on numero uno! Since you feel justified, your enemy votes for the flesh as well; and there you go—two against one! Your own heart will lie to you. It will say, Hey, you're not so bad; others do a lot worse or just one time every now and then won't hurt. Yes it will! Don't you know the enemy planted those thoughts in your head? He wants you to ignore the warning bells that go off when you do or think things that you wouldn't do or think if God were standing next to you.

Respect your father (God)! He loves you; but if He has to take you out to the woodshed for your own good, He will! Please don't make Him do that. It's going to hurt! He constantly gives protection in the heavenly realms for those who are called according to His purpose. What if you're not living according to your Godly purpose? Does any of your behavior fit outside of God's purpose? You bet! Take that trash out! Your father can (and will) remove His protection and blessing from you if your rebellion continues. He has many promises of protection and guidance in His Word. So, if you're not following His lead, you risk the terrible consequences of being open to attack. Satan can get the permission—and he has to—to go after you. He can and will pursue you like a hound on a rabbit.

Where are you in your relationship with God right now? I don't mean five years ago, five months ago, or even five days ago, but right now? Where would you rate it at this moment on a scale of one to ten? Be honest! Do you know that He wants a ten relationship with us, that He desires to be so close to us in fellowship and friendship that He sent Jesus to take our punishment for all the sins we have ever or will ever commit in order to have the right relationship with Him? You can be as close to God as you want to be; it's all up to you. But you have to want that enough to forsake all other "lovers"; you have to make Him the only "Lover of your Soul." What is it in your life that keeps you from that relationship right now? I will tell you from personal experience—it's not worth it!

Right now, bow your head and ask God to forgive you for all the things you've allowed to become more important in your life than Him. Ask Him to forgive you of any and all sin that you have allowed to come in and made excuses for. Tell Him you want Him to be your Best Friend. Now thank Him for doing that in Jesus' name! If you mean it, then you have started on the right path back to healing of discouragement in your life.

Second, spend time hearing from God. Read His "love letters" to you. Did you know that the Bible is God's personal love letter to each of us? The more we read it, the more we see and understand that God has a perfect plan for our lives, which is better and more fulfilling than any plan you or I could come up with! Read as much about Jesus as you can; read His words and become acquainted with His heart! It is full of compassion, mercy, and love!

Third, spend time "talking" to Him. We call that prayer. Many of you think prayer is some formal, stuffy way of talking to an impersonal God who might be listening. No, talking to God is like talking to your best friend! He is your best friend! Talk to Him all day long—you don't have to get on your knees every time and say something formal! Throughout the day keep a continual stream of chatter going to Him as if He were right there with you in the car, the grocery store, at work, in the kitchen, or wherever—because He is! Yes, you need to set aside time to get on your knees and focus just on Him, but He loves the "small talk" too; and as you cultivate this relationship with Him, you will begin to sense His presence and direction in your life throughout the day. You will begin to gather strength and confidence as never before!

And fourth, learn to be in a state of constant praise. The scripture tells us that "God inhabits the praises of His people." Think about that! When you and I begin to praise God, He shows up! Praise Him throughout the day—in your car, at work, and when you get up in the morning. If you will cultivate a heart of praise, discouragement will find it hard to take root in your life.

Are things hard or difficult right now? Then ask Him to come into the situation and give you the wisdom and knowledge to get through it. Ask Him to intervene and bring a miracle where there seems to be no hope. Then acknowledge that you don't know how He's going to do it; but since He is in control, you are going to praise Him ahead of time for the answer!

I want to encourage you in this area of your life. We all get discouraged at times, but God wants us to learn how to beat this enemy of our souls and to live victorious lives! If you are discouraged, then all you can think about is you and your own situation. But if you will rise above it, you will open up an entirely new area of your life to where God can begin to use you in a powerful way to bring about change and restoration, not only in your life, but in the lives of others you come into contact with.

Chapter 27

Another thing I learned is how to have compassion for those who are sick even though I may not understand the sickness. There are people all around us going through things we don't quite understand because we've never really experienced them ourselves. A lot of times we are quick to judge or give our opinion about their situation based on our own limited knowledge. Or, maybe, we have had some similar experience, so, all of a sudden, we become an expert on the subject. No two situations are ever exactly alike—each person is different in his personality and prior experiences leading up to whatever they are going through. I learned this lesson the hard way many years ago and now have watched as I myself have been the one being judged. Let me share a story of an experience that happened to me several years ago.

Before going into the ministry in 1995, I was an Elder at a local church. I remember on a particular Sunday morning I was standing in the foyer before the service, when an elderly couple walked in. They seemed to be upset about something, so I went up to them and asked them if there was a problem. They said that their little dog had died the day before, and then they began to cry. I patted them on the back, told them everything would be all right, and said they could get another dog! I also thought to myself, What's the big deal!? It's just a dog! I grew up on a farm and had seen many animals die and had even had to kill some of them. I thought to myself, they'll get another dog! Then I went about my normal duties for the rest of the morning without thinking another thing about it.

Several years later I was pastoring a vibrant, growing church. Things were going well and life seemed great. Then one Saturday afternoon I was getting ready to go to the church and participate in a leadership meeting. I parked my car in the front yard close to the front door of the house so that I could make a quick run to the car later since it had been raining off and on throughout the day. It was time for me to go, and there was a typical Florida downpour occurring. I ran from the front porch and got into my car as quickly as possible. Then I started the engine and waited for a few moments. I always waited because we had an old, grey tomcat we called Smokey, and he liked to get under my car all the time and just lie there. Whenever I would start the engine, Smokey would come running out. So I started my car and waited. Since I saw no Smokey, I backed out onto the street. All of a sudden I saw movement in the corner of my eye, so I looked over into the grass where I had just backed out. There was Smokey—he had been under the car the whole time and had not come out because of the downpour. I had backed over his head, and he was flopping around on the ground in the front yard! I was struck with immediate horror at what had occurred!

I pulled back into the yard as quickly as possible and, oblivious to the rain, got out and ran over to him. I picked him up and took him to the shed in the backyard and stayed with him until he died. I knew I couldn't let my two oldest boys see him in that condition because it would have crushed them. Smokey had been part of our blended family longer than I had! When he finally passed, I went into the house and told the boys what had happened. They were grief stricken, but so was I!

That old cat had become a valuable member of our family, in a pet-sort-of-way; and I was the guy who took him out! I cried and cried; then remembered I still had a meeting to go to at the church, so I climbed back in my car and began driving to the church. I was crying so hard that I ran a four way stop sign without realizing it until I was already through it by about fifty feet or more! Thank goodness there were no other cars pulling through at that moment!

As I continued to drive, I began praying through my tears and my grief. I asked God, Why did you let Smokey die! And if he had to die, why did it have to be me!? Why couldn't you just let him run out onto the highway and get hit by a total stranger, so I wouldn't have to carry that guilt and grief of being the one who did it? No sooner had I asked the questions, when the Holy Spirit whispered deep into my soul and brought back a picture in my mind so vividly that it seemed as if it happened only moments before. Remember when the older couple came into the church long ago, on that Sunday morning, after having just lost their little dog? Remember how you responded to them in a way that lacked any compassion and sympathy for how they felt that morning? Now you understand the pain they experienced that day, and you will never respond to grief the same way again.

It was just a whisper, but it was as clear as a bell to me! He had allowed me to learn a valuable lesson, that is, that we don't know what someone is going through until we ourselves have been there. Therefore, deal with each situation in a way that gives others the benefit of the doubt without casting judgment on them. Show compassion to those who are hurting around you, even though you may not understand their pain or particular set of circumstances. Try to see them through the eyes of Jesus. It doesn't mean that you are excusing known sin in their lives.

I would never suggest overlooking and condoning known sin in a person's life. It simply means we have compassion for their situation and seek to find help, answers, and a way back to restoration—back to God, not to gossip and judgment.

Matthew 7:1-5 (NLT) says, "Do not judge others, and you will not be judged.[2] For you will be treated as you treat others. The standard you use in judging is the standard by which you will be judged.[3] And why worry about a speck in your friend's eye when you have a log in your own? [4] How can you think of saying to your friend, Let me help you get rid of that speck in your eye, when you can't see past the log in your own eye? [5] Hypocrite! First get rid of the log in your own eye; then you will see well enough to deal with the speck in your friend's eye."

I saw this principle played out many times during the year and a half of my depression. Some said to me, I had depression and got over it; you can too if you want to badly enough!

Another said, Just get over it and quit using it as an excuse! Others would say, You should just "get on with it" and get over it! Several of these individuals were from my congregation. They were ones I had shown compassion to during difficult situations they had faced! This both surprised and discouraged me in my hour of deepest need.

Many times we face people suffering from conditions that we have very little personal experience with, so we struggle to know what to say. But depression is such a common illness now and is on the rise around the world at such an alarming rate, that chances are you have someone right now who is a family member or friend suffering with it. How are you responding? People can and do recover from depression, but it is of great importance that you take the time to pray and give them positive support, not criticism and a judgmental spirit.

Judging others is a form of pride. We look at our own store of knowledge, put together a few facts and figures, and then come up with some sort of answer or solution to the problem, as we see it. Most of the time it is the wrong answer or solution; but because of pride, we refuse to be corrected. God, however, has specific consequences for those whose pride leads them to this false view of themselves.

Proverbs 16:18 (NIV): "Pride goes before destruction, a haughty spirit before a fall."

Ecclesiastes 7:8 (NIV): "The end of a matter is better than its beginning, and patience is better than pride."

When you judge someone, you have chosen to take on yourself the responsibility for making the correct judgment. Only God truly knows the heart of a man!

1 Samuel 16:7 (NLT): "But the Lord said to Samuel, 'Don't judge by his appearance or height, for I have rejected him.' The Lord doesn't see things the way you see them. People judge by outward appearance, but the Lord looks at the heart."

After we judge, we make matters worse by believing in our judgment of the situation or circumstance. We have looked at the evidence, so it must be right! There just couldn't be any other conclusion! I must be right, even though I've never really been where they are!

What most people don't see is that judging often leads to suffering, not only for the person you have judged, but eventually, also for you. God wants you to see others through the eyes of love—that is how we will be judged.

James 2:12-13 (NLT): "¹² So whatever you say or whatever you do, remember that you will be judged by the law that sets you free. ¹³ There will be no mercy for those who have not shown mercy to others. But if you have been merciful, God will be merciful when he judges you."

In writing the story of my depression, it was my hope and prayer that it would help and encourage many others who are currently experiencing something similar to what I went through. A lot of you have contacted me to let me know that it has helped you in some way. But I also knew that by writing this account, it would open the doors for some to be critical and judgmental. You can't share some of the intimate details of your life without opening yourself up to be examined and ultimately judged. There's just no way around it. But what I now understand is this: the risk of being transparent and on the critical end of someone's words is worth it if through the experience being told, it gives hope to even one person.

In several instances recorded in scripture, Jesus looked on the crowd with compassion. I used to tell my congregation on a regular basis that each Sunday the churches all across America are filled with hurting people. All of us have problems. All of us have pain and disappointments. Each of us will go through trials and temptations on a regular basis, no matter what our station in life is. So the next time you begin to be critical of someone, remember that you might find yourself in that same situation someday. How would you want others to feel about you and treat you? Would you want criticism and judgment, or would you desire compassion, mercy, grace, and especially, the prayers and helping hands of others?

Chapter 28

Life is tough sometimes. We are not promised a rosy, happy-go-lucky today; but we are promised an Eternity where we will have no more sorrow, pain, sickness, or death! I'm not proud of the stuff I did while I was going through the depression, but I'm not going to grovel because of my mistakes either. There are those who will throw your past up to you in order to justify how they act in the present. There is then the temptation to relive all of your mistakes, sins, and heartaches. Don't do it! It doesn't matter whether they believe in you, trust you, or even acknowledge God's intervention, forgiveness, and healing in your life. What matters is what has taken place between you and your Creator!

God is a God of forgiveness, healing, and mercy. Not until we have gone down the road ourselves, can we see how unlike Christ it is to be unforgiving and without mercy. God is a God of second, third, fourth, and many more chances; yet we will hold something over someone else's head for years without any regard for the miracle wrought in their lives. Instead of rejoicing with them over the victory they have received in their battle against the enemy, we continue to whisper and act as if they have committed the unpardonable sin! Lord help us and have mercy on us!

I didn't realize to what extent we do this to each other until I went through it myself. Wow! Sinners have no problem accepting someone who has messed up and is now putting the pieces back together again. In fact, they can identify; and it gives them a sense of hope for their own predicaments. But we, the Church of Jesus Christ—-now that's a different story! Why do we go ahead and shoot our own wounded? Why are we more lacking in mercy than those outside of the church? Do you really want to know why? If you're serious, read on. If not, stop right here.

Here's the reason why: people have trouble forgiving others because they don't know how to be forgiving of themselves when they mess up, do wrong, aren't perfect,

117

or whatever the situation may be. When we see the sin or mistakes of others, we also see their reflection in ourselves. Many of the things they have done we have done or at least have thought about doing and are capable of doing at any given moment! 1 Corinthians 10:12 (NIV) says, "So, if you think you are standing firm, be careful that you don't fall!"

If we were to examine all of the times we have sinned, made mistakes, or even hurt others, we would find that we have no reason to hold others to a higher standard than we hold ourselves. Romans 3:23 tells us that "ALL have sinned and fallen short of God's glorious ideal or standard." That includes you and me. You and I are not exempt.

Hold in your left or right hand a very heavy book. Extend your arm with the book in it. How long can you hold that position before YOU MUST LET GO? How long do you want to hold onto that resentment, anger, unforgiveness, or even pride? It is pride that says to others, Thank God I'm not like them! It is pride that says, "I would never do anything like that!" Be careful! The enemy is already crouching at your door!

If you don't let go of your pride, learn to forgive, and show compassion and mercy to others, physical hurt, illness, or pain will start growing in your own body and soul. Letting go and forgiving will bring back the joy and happiness you need in your life and will release you, along with the other person, to move forward and have a productive life in the Kingdom of God. Who is so perfect, anyway, other than God? If God, the Creator of all, is so forgiving; and Jesus died on the cross for our transgressions—to erase all of our mess-ups; and if He forgives us, who are we not to forgive?

Pride is such an ugly word, yet we wear it every day in some form or fashion. Pride comes in the form of criticism and unforgiveness. How many times have you ever looked at something that someone else has done, and said, I'd never do that? Look at what Jesus has to say about it:

Matthew 6:14-15 (NIV)—"14For if you forgive men when they sin against you, your heavenly Father will *also forgive you. ¹⁵But if you do not forgive men their sins, your Father will not forgive your sins."*

Luke 17:3-4 (NIV)—"³So watch yourselves. "If your brother sins, rebuke him, and if he repents, forgive him. ⁴If he sins against you seven times in a day, and seven times comes back to you and says, 'I repent,' forgive him."

Listen to what the Apostle Paul said to the church at Colossae: *Colossians 3:12-14 (NIV)—*

"¹²Therefore, as God's chosen people, holy and dearly loved, clothe yourselves with compassion, kindness, humility, gentleness and patience. ¹³Bear with each other and forgive whatever grievances you may have against one another. Forgive as the Lord forgave you. ¹⁴And over all these virtues put on love, which binds them all together in perfect unity."

Put on love. "Love" is an action word. Love is shown in what we do, not what we say. Do you remember the old adage, "Actions speak louder than words"? Listen to what the scriptures say:

1 Corinthians 13:1-3 (NIV)—"¹If I speak in the tongues of men and of angels, but have not love, I am only a resounding gong or a clanging cymbal. ²If I have the gift of prophecy and can fathom all mysteries and all knowledge, and if I have a faith that can move mountains, but have not love, I am nothing.

³If I give all I possess to the poor and surrender my body to the flames, but have not love, I gain nothing."

Don't tell me you have the love of God if you ignore me, or continue to talk about me, or fail to rejoice when I have been delivered and set free. The religion that is being practiced is then nothing more than a form of Godliness with no power attached to it at all. If God's love truly abides, we will have forgiveness and mercy on others and our lives will then bear fruit for the Kingdom of God.

Galatians 5:13-15 (NIV)—"[13] You, my brothers, were called to be free. But do not use your freedom to indulge the sinful nature; rather, serve one another in love. [14] The entire law is summed up in a single command: "Love your neighbor as yourself." [15] If you keep on biting and devouring each other, watch out or you will be destroyed by each other."

Are you ready to be free? Then forgive. Love others as God does, and only then will your life begin to bear lasting fruit for the Kingdom of God!

Chapter 29

There's a fire burning deep within me that wants to get out. Let me explain. When I was fifteen years old, a sophomore in high school, I started attending a private Christian High School in Kentucky during the fall of 1972. The only reason I wanted to go there was that, at the time, there was a girl from my church in Marion, Ohio, whom I was crazy about. She was attending there, so I thought in order to be closer to her and see her every day, I would attend there also and as a result be able to develop a closer relationship with her. Boy, what a surprise was waiting for me when I got there! Not only did I find out that the boys and girls could not interact at any level, even talk to each other; but I also found out she was crazy about one of the guys who was a senior! Talk about "bummed out"!

So I settled into high school life there, playing different sports, going to classes, and making new friends, except this was different. This was a Christian high school. There was no swearing, drinking, drugs, or even the remotest chance of kissing a girl, let alone sex! But I was into sports anyway, so none of that was something that consumed me. Give me a basketball, a bat and glove, a tennis racket, and a football; and I was in my own little heaven! But there was also something else different; most of the kids there were Christians, except for me and a few others. Oh, I was raised in a Christian home and had attended church since I was four years old, but that Christian stuff just wasn't for me! It was for the old "fuddy duddies" in the churches I had grown up in!

I still remember the night my Mom got saved in a little Nazarene Church in Upper Sandusky, Ohio. As I have said, I was four at the time. I remember that on the way home from church that night my mom threw her cigarettes out the car window. That started a whole family thing of church twice every Sunday and mid-week service every Wednesday from that time forward! Eventually my Dad also got saved, so then we really were a church going family! So here I was, raised in a Christian home, but with a hard heart. Over the years I had rejected Christ, service after service, camp meeting after camp meeting.

At fifteen I had developed a really hard heart. I wanted nothing of the Christianity I had seen in many of the people I had gone to church with over the years. I've often wondered why, but in recent years I have come to believe there were a couple of reasons. For one, I didn't want to be like the Christians I had come to know, who ran the churches we attended. I saw harshness to their way of life and many times a lack of love in their dealings with others. They also made it a point to say that they were happy, but they just didn't look like it or act like it. Many of them I would consider "mean Christians." I know that is an oxymoron, but it was the truth! It is not to say that there weren't some who were kind over the years, but they were far and few between! I also saw a lot of petty fighting and fussing over things that seemed so trivial and nonessential, and I wanted no part of it!

Second of all, I thought that once you were a Christian, you couldn't have fun anymore. I saw God as a big bully in heaven, ready to hit you with a club if you got Him mad enough! That was the "gospel" that was preached and lived with many I had grown up with. So I was content to go to church and let everyone else get saved, but it wasn't for me! Then something happened at school; they had a fall revival! And all of us students were required to attend every night of it for the entire week! All the sporting events were shut down and church was the main menu! I was extremely unhappy about this turn of events. That really threw a monkey wrench into my plans!

The revival started, and each night there was an altar call for students to come forward and receive Christ or for them to seek a deeper walk with God. Many were seeking God's call and plan for their lives. Boy was I sweating it! I saw many students receive Jesus as their personal Savior. I also witnessed several classmates receive the call of God on their lives for the mission field or ministry of some sort. But I was determined I was not going to give in; and the more I resisted, the more miserable I got!

Our boys' dormitory had been transformed into a house of prayer. Students were attending Bible studies and spending hours in prayer without the prompting of the faculty and staff. I was amazed! But I held out until the last night! By this time, every student on campus, over two hundred in all, had received Christ or been set free in some way except for me. The last night came; and I remember that as the altar call was given, many students came up to me and asked if I wanted to go forward and receive Christ. People all over the auditorium were praying—many of them for me! Finally, so miserable I could hardly stand it, I stepped out into the aisle and went forward. The altar was so full of people praying and getting victory over all sorts of junk in their lives that I had to kneel at the end of the pew on the front row.

I can take you to that spot today and show you where I kneeled in prayer. That moment is as clear as the light of day, because when I knelt, I asked Jesus to forgive me of all of my sins and become my Lord and Savior! All of a sudden, I felt as if a ton of bricks had just been lifted from my heart and life; and at fifteen years old, in September of 1972, my name was written in the Lamb's Book of Life! Hallelujah! Praise God! I was free! Jesus had saved me! I became a Child of the King of kings and Lord of lords that day! I immediately fell in love with Jesus and wanted to serve Him!

Then a peculiar thing happened to me a couple of months later. I was rooming with a couple of other guys in the dormitory. It was late at night, and all three of us were asleep in our bunks. I was on the top bunk, and in the middle of my sleep I heard a voice speak to me. It very simply called my name—David. Have you ever had a dream so vivid that it woke you up in the middle of the night? That's what happened to me! I immediately found myself wide awake thinking one of the guys wanted to talk. I checked, but they were all soundly asleep. So I lay back down and was thinking about what had just occurred when I heard it again—David!

I don't know if anyone else in the room would have heard it if they had been awake, but it was an audible voice to me. I immediately sensed it was God wanting to speak to me. It didn't frighten me at all. In fact, I felt a peace about it. So I lay there and quietly told the Lord I was listening. He then spoke to my spirit with a message as clear as a bell and told me He wanted me to preach the Gospel. I simply said, Yes, Lord, and with peace in my heart, rolled over and went back to sleep!

You can believe it or not; it doesn't matter to me. I knew nothing at the time of the story in the Bible about Eli and Samuel. I studied that later in Bible College and thought it was really neat that I had had such a similar experience, confirming even more God's call for my life. I know what God has called me to do, and since that time I have had a longing and a burning desire to see souls won to Christ!

Fast forward—I eventually received a bachelor's degree in Religion with a double major in Ministry and Missions. Then I went on to Morehead State University where I received another bachelor's degree in Education with a major in Geography and a minor in Religion. I have been involved in all types of church work since then: Music Minister, Sunday School Superintendent, Sunday School teacher, Elder, board member, and so forth. I have been a school teacher for over thirty years, as well as a coach of junior high and high school basketball teams along the way. And I have also been through a failed first marriage, children, and grandchildren. Eventually I started and pastored a church for thirteen years. Now you come to this present time in my life. You have heard how I battled depression and how God ultimately healed my life. But now comes the time to answer the question, Why?

Chapter 30

Why did God allow this all to happen? We all have our theories, but the Bible tells us that we are constantly being tried and tested. 1 Peter 1:6 (NIV) says: "⁶In this you greatly rejoice, though now for a little while you may have had to suffer grief in all kinds of trials."

These times come in order for God's glory to be seen even in the worst of circumstances. They are times for us to grow in our trust and our relationship with Christ. We are being constantly conformed to His image. The more we realize we need Him and call out to Him in our struggles, the more we see Him work and see His will and purpose worked out in our lives. Let me explain on a personal level.

Years before the depression overtook me, God had been moving in my life in a powerful way. About ten years ago I began to feel I needed a more intimate walk with God, so I began to really seek His face and ask Him to draw me closer. Be careful what you ask for! In order to be more like Christ, we have to become less like ourselves. Spiritually we have to die to things we want and what we want to do and let Christ through His Holy Spirit live more through us.

Romans 8:12-14 (NIV)—"¹²Therefore, brothers, we have an obligation—but it is not to the sinful nature, to live according to it. ¹³For if you live according to the sinful nature, you will die; but if by the Spirit you put to death the misdeeds of the body, you will live, ¹⁴because those who are led by the Spirit of God are sons of God."

The flesh only produces more flesh, and the Spirit produces more of the Spirit. The more we yield to the Spirit of God in our lives, the more we see how ugly the flesh is. Then we have to make a choice—continue letting the Spirit cut away at the flesh or stop and try to be content where we are spiritually. In other words, if you want to grow and be more like Jesus, the more of you Christ is going to strip away. That's a good thing, but it's painful!

When I asked God to draw me closer, He began to put people in my path who could help accomplish that—both good and bad ones! I started meeting with another pastor in town to pray and seek the things of God. Mike Brown was the pastor at Dunklin Memorial Camp at the time. He is now the pastor of "The Gathering," a vibrant Spirit filled church in Okeechobee, Florida. Dunklin Church and Camp is a place where drug and alcohol addictions are ministered to. It is a place where many are set free and then released back into the world to continue their lives under the power of God. Pastor Mike Brown is a man I respected greatly, and still do. So I went to him, and we began a time of partnering together in prayer.

I was so hungry at the time—hungry to have more of God in my life and hungry to win souls at an even greater level than I had ever done before! I had this longing down deep and nothing I did would satisfy it. I knew I was saved. I knew that God was using the ministry we had started to win many souls to Christ, but I wasn't satisfied. There was something more and I was missing it!

As we met to pray, I expressed to him the frustration I was feeling. I told him that I didn't know what the frustration was all about. He asked me if I had ever received the Baptism of the Holy Spirit. I said had not, but that I had heard of it and knew it was in the Bible. I had even studied it at Bible College, but I told him I had always been taught it was a false doctrine and that people who practiced speaking in tongues were not real Christians. But I also let him know that I didn't believe those judgments because my mom was a Christian and was filled with the Spirit when I was a teen-ager. I knew she spoke in tongues on a regular basis. I just didn't think it was for me. I was confused about it but willing to seek it if it truly was from God and for everybody.

That day he laid his hands on my head and prayed over me. He asked God to baptize me in the Spirit and give me the gift of tongues. He also prayed over me in tongues. I was very curious about the whole ordeal and listened intently as he prayed. It was the first time anything like that had ever happened to me! When he was done, I thanked him and then went home. I felt no power surge or any extra feeling, but I will tell you that the next day when I preached, there was something different. I couldn't put my finger on it, but something had changed!

That started a mini-revival at the church. People began coming to the altar in larger numbers for all sorts of reasons. Many people were being saved. I was anointing others with oil and praying over them for healing and watching many be healed of all kinds of afflictions, including cancer, tumors, arthritis, migraines, and back problems, with many of these being authenticated by the individuals' doctors!

The church also experienced a spike in growth. Complete strangers would show up on Sunday morning at the front door with tears in their eyes. They would tell us that as they were driving by, they felt a pull to drive into the parking lot and come in. They would begin crying the moment they got in the parking lot, but didn't know why. Many people told us of how they had begun crying as soon as they entered the church grounds and the building! I knew what it was! It was the Holy Spirit who was drawing them and softening their hearts so they would receive the Gospel!

Week after the week the altar was full. There were times when so many people were kneeling that it was three and four deep, and I had to step over people just to get to the ones to pray with who the Spirit was directing me to. Linda was also ministering around the altar with people at that time, along with a prayer team I had to organize and teach how to pray with seekers. What an incredible move of God it was! To lead souls to Christ and see the weight of sins lifted from their lives; to see someone with cancer completely healed and restored; to see marriages restored by the power of God; to see hope in the eyes of someone who had no hope—these are beautiful experiences. I didn't really preach any differently or feel any different from before, but now I see that it is not who we are, but who He is! When God's anointing is present in the life of a believer, it will produce much fruit for the Kingdom of God!

But something was still missing. You might think, Are you crazy?! God is doing all that and yet you are still seeking more?! Absolutely—I don't want to settle for good. I want God's BEST for my life! We know when something down deep is still telling us that there's more. I had this fire in my belly, which wouldn't go away. I had this ache in my heart, which kept telling me we had just touched the surface of what God wanted to do, and I was still missing something. But what was it?

Five or six years ago I was doing some Christmas shopping for my wife. I went to Vero Beach that Sunday afternoon to shop at the Indian River Mall. We didn't hold a Sunday night service, so it wasn't imperative for me to get back at any certain time. I did my shopping and then the announcement was made that the mall would be closing in fifteen minutes. It was closing at 7:00 p.m.! Why was it closing so early during the Christmas season!? I got my packages and left the store. As I was traveling west to go home on Route 60, I noticed a sign on the left-hand side, which had the name "Pastor Buddy" on it. I had seen it many times before and was always curious as to what kind of service went on in that big metal building. I always wondered who in the world this Pastor Buddy guy could be!

Since Linda wasn't expecting me home until late, I decided to go on in. I slipped in the back and sat down. The music was playing. It was the same things we were doing at our church—a full praise and worship band with the same songs. Everything seemed the same except there were a lot more people. Then Pastor Buddy got up to preach. That night he was speaking on the Baptism of the Spirit and with the evidence of speaking in tongues. Good! I was still very curious about the whole thing.

As he began to preach, that familiar ache began to come over me again. I made up my mind I was going to go up front if there was an altar call! At the end of the message, Pastor

Buddy said if anyone wanted to be baptized in the Holy Spirit and receive the gift of tongues, then they should come forward. I thought to myself, You are completely incognito! Not a soul in this place knows me, which means they don't know I'm a minister either! That was a good thing. I just wanted to fly under the radar, get this Baptism thing if that's what I needed, and then get out of there!

There were people across the front of the church who were there to pray with those who came forward. They were facing the congregation. I stepped into the aisle and made my way to the front. Another line had formed across the front facing the prayer team. There were several people to my left and several all the way down to my right who had also come forward. I really didn't know what to expect next. This was all new to me. But I had a sense of anticipation—could this be the night that I might finally fill this void, which had nagged at me over and over for years?

One of the men started toward me to minister to me. He got about three feet away when all of a sudden he stopped, threw both of his hands up in the air and said, "Whoa!" He looked at me and said, "You're a minister of the Gospel aren't you? You're a servant of the Lord!" I was shocked! How did he know? It was then I realized that this was totally uncharted water for me. I told him I was; he looked at me and said, "What can I do for you?" He seemed to be wondering why a minister needed to be prayed over, rather than my praying over him. I simply told him that I wanted everything God had for me, that I wanted more of God in my life. So, he had me lift my hands; and he started praying for me, alternating between English and speaking in tongues. I was totally receptive that night, but nothing seemed to happen again. After awhile of praying and crying out to God, I thanked him and left. I went home and told Linda what had happened but soon settled back into a routine again.

One more incident occurred a couple of years later. I met Roy Gardner, a missionary to Australia. He and his wife, Barbara, had become friends with Linda and me. They owned a place north of Okeechobee called the Golden Wattle Ranch. It was a place where missionaries and ministers from around the world could go in order to get away and spend time with God. I loved to go out there. There were even times when Linda would take some of the ladies from the church for seminars and retreats. Roy had become a mentor to me and often prayed with me about the ministry. He felt strongly that ministers needed mentoring. He felt they needed someone they confide in and pray with, knowing their concerns would stay confidential.

One Sunday, Roy and Barbara came to the church to give their testimony. They had felt God calling them back to Australia, so they sold the ranch and were getting ready to move. I remember vividly what happened next. Before the morning service started, I was standing in the church kitchen behind the serving counter. Roy was on the other side of the counter having a cup of coffee and talking with me. I was feeling that familiar, nagging feeling strongly that morning—that hunger and thirst for a deeper walk with God and the feeling that I was still missing out on something. I told Roy about it. I told him that I was envious that he could sell everything and move across the world in order to preach the Gospel.

I'll never forget his response—"Dave, he said, "have you ever considered that your work here at this church may be done? Have you considered that maybe God wants you to minister somewhere else or to start another church?" Something welled up inside of me! Tears began to flow from the corners of my eyes as I told him that I didn't see how any of that could happen but that I would go anywhere the Lord wanted me to go and minister the Gospel to whomever He wanted me to minister to!

That unsettling feeling never left me; even up until the time I went into depression, I felt that God had a wonderful plan for my life, a mission He wanted me to be a part of. Seeing no way to accomplish anything like what Roy and Barbara were doing, I put it into the back of my mind and set about trying to be the best minister I could be. I figured

I would just try to bloom where God had planted me; and if there was more, then He was going to have to make it happen. I went along like that for a few more years, and then the bottom fell out. I started a year and a half of hell on earth.

Chapter 31

Let's fast forward beyond the depression. You've read the story; now I'll tackle the question of why God allowed me to go through this. There were several reasons, in no particular order of significance. First, I believe God wanted me to grow. I know that sounds crazy, but I believe He wanted to continue cutting away areas of my life in the flesh, and help me to walk more in step with the Spirit.

1 Peter 4:12-13 (NIV) says: "12Dear friends, do not be surprised at the painful trial you are suffering, as though something strange were happening to you. 13But rejoice that you participate in the sufferings of Christ, so that you may be overjoyed when his glory is revealed."

Peter calls them painful trials that we suffer and says we are to rejoice in them! I rejoice now, but I sure didn't rejoice while I was going through my trial! I look back on it all now and see that God was getting me into a position to break me down in order to begin rebuilding me. When you get so low that the only way is up, then God can start peeling away the layers. And peel away He did! I was a broken vessel on the potter's wheel. He wanted to reshape me and mold me into something different and new.

Jeremiah 18:3-4 (NIV) says:"" So I went down to the potter's house, and I saw him working at the wheel. 4 But the pot he was shaping from the clay was marred in his hands; so the potter formed it into another pot, shaping it as seemed best to him."

Even though I was saved, He wanted to transform the way I thought, the way I viewed and did ministry, how I preached, and what I preached about. It wasn't that what I did was all wrong. It was that I was just working on four cylinders and not the full eight. God wanted me to be able to reach people in a way that would have never been possible before.

Romans 12:1-2 (NIV) says: "1Therefore, I urge you, brothers, in view of God's mercy, to offer your bodies as living sacrifices, holy and pleasing to God—this is your spiritual act of worship. [2]Do not conform any longer to the pattern of this world, but be transformed by the renewing of your mind. Then you will be able to test and approve what God's will is—his good, pleasing and perfect will."

I see the world through different eyes now. I see ministry through a whole new lens. My preaching will never be the same. What is the biggest difference in me? That's the second thing. The biggest change in me that came about as a result of the depression is that I finally received the Baptism of the Holy Spirit! What a tremendous gift! Hallelujah! Let me tell you how it happened and the results of it.

In Chapter 16 I wrote about the Men's Encounter I attended four weeks after my initial healing. One of the parts I didn't relate was the special service on Sunday at the retreat. We had gathered together that morning, and all of us sat in a large circle in the room. A couple of the leaders were in the middle of the room and did a teaching on the Baptism of the Holy Spirit, with the initial sign being that you would speak in an unknown language that the Spirit gave you.

By this time in the retreat I had had so many issues of the past dealt with and removed that I was ready! So the leaders called us to come and stand in the middle of the room with them. We were paired with different facilitators, sometimes two or three, who laid hands on us and prayed over us asking God for the Baptism of the Holy Spirit. I remember I was standing there and hearing the room just swell to a crescendo of sound that was so beautiful! Not only were men praying in English, but this groundswell of languages I had never heard before began to permeate the room. Although the experience was different from what I was used to, it all seemed so natural and brought a sense of peace and yet incredible power with it.

I was awestruck! Almost every man in the room had his hands raised in prayer and praise to the Almighty. Tears were streaming freely and openly. Every once in a while I would hear a shout of victory go up from several men as another man from the retreat would be Baptized in the Spirit and begin speaking in an unknown prayer language. It was absolutely beautiful! I had my hands raised and was in earnest prayer to God. I was sobbing by now and truly broken before the Lord of all Creation. My hands were in the air, and I was crying out in praise and adoration, at the same time asking God to come in His might and power and fill me with His Spirit! Time flew by. When you are in God's presence, everything else seems so insignificant.

About half an hour into it, something very dramatic happened. I had a vision. It was as clear as you reading this page right now. You may not believe in visions, but I can assure you that they are real. The whole ceiling and sky peeled back, and I saw something happening; it was like viewing a movie. I was looking down into the middle of the church I had pastored. All of the people were in the middle of the church, and they were going around and around in a big circle. This big crowd just kept going around and around and around. I could see and sense that they were lost and confused.

Directly in the middle of the circle I saw one who stood out from the rest. He was going in circles also but was trying to lead them. He was shuffling his feet as he moved, but he was moving very slow and not getting very far. He was looking up, but with a lost, confused, and stricken look on his face. It was one of the men who had been instrumental in getting rid of me, forcing me to resign. Then, just as clear as a bell, the Spirit spoke to me. He said, "Pray for them. They are sheep without a shepherd, and they don't know where they are going. They are confused and lost."

I was horrified! Here I was, praying to God with all of my heart; and right in the middle of it God shows me this vision of my former congregation in deep distress and need! Did you ever feel as if your heart was being ripped from you? I began to weep and weep and weep. I grabbed one of the guys who had been praying with me and hugged him as I somehow sobbed out what had just happened. My heart was torn! I was in agony! We began to pray, and we didn't stop until God lifted the burden. Needless to say, even though I had been praying for the Baptism of the Holy Spirit and continued awhile longer doing that, it wasn't to be at that time.

Let me interject into the story and tell you why I believe the Lord showed me this vision. First of all, it was wrong for those involved to force my resignation. Had they waited on God a little longer, I feel sure it was just a matter of a short period of time before I would have done it on my own anyway. I knew I was sick and needed God's help and healing. But I needed to come to the place where I made the decision. I also needed the opportunity to leave with some dignity and honor. You don't take the one who started the church, was the only minister it ever had, and force him out the door. Not only that, it was wrong of them to insist that I get everything out of my office in a timely manner or have it removed by them! Is that the respect you give someone who has poured his life into the people of that church and community?

What they did was usurp the spiritual authority God had placed on me to lead the congregation. When you take the ministry from someone whom God has placed and anointed for that position, you take for yourself what can only be given. You now are in a position God did not give you. You are no longer operating under the authority, power, and anointing of God's Holy Spirit. And believe me, the anointing is everything! Without the anointing you will not bear fruit. You may be a good speaker and say some good things, but the anointing brings life-changing power into the words you speak and bears fruit for the Kingdom of God!

You can try all the gimmicks in the world, but you will not bear fruit for the Kingdom. You will eventually become a country club–a friendly group of people who like to hang out together, but who bear no lasting fruit for the Kingdom. What you take by force you must now keep by force. You have now left the congregation vulnerable without their shepherd. People will scatter, and many will not return to any fold. But what God gives, He anoints and maintains.

God tells us through His word and gives examples of this principle: we are not to touch God's anointed. When Saul sinned and God then anointed David to be the next king of Israel, there were many times David could have risen up against Saul and even slain him; but he was respectful of the choice God had made and waited until many years later when Saul finally died. He refused not only to touch and harm, but also to speak against God's anointed. Sometimes we feel we can do a better job than the guy in charge; but just remember, if you touch God's anointed, you will pay a high price for it. It is the Lord's responsibility to remove them and discipline them, not ours. I would recommend that each of you read John Bevere's book Undercover. These principles are laid out scripturally so that one can understand. As I said, I didn't receive the baptism at the retreat, but about three weeks later something happened in the middle of the night.

Chapter 32

Another reason why God allowed me to go through a serious depression, I believe, was to get me into a place where I would be receptive to ALL God had for me. The Baptism of the Holy Spirit is at the top of that list. As you have read, I prayed and searched for years but without finding what I was looking and longing for. I didn't know that Baptism of the Holy Spirit was what I was missing in my heart, life, and spiritual walk. Three weeks after the Men's Encounter and the experience with the vision He had given me, I had an encounter with God that altered the entire course of my life and changed my ministry forever.

I woke up around 1:00 in the morning and couldn't get back to sleep. I was still reveling in the afterglow of more than a month of divine healing; so I decided to go outside on the front porch, sit on the bench, and spend time praying to the Lord. As I began to pray, I sensed His presence all around me and in me. I began to praise Him for all He had done—for His forgiveness, for His mercy, for the healing I had received, for setting me free from bondages I had been victim to all of my life. This went on for about twenty minutes or so. Then in the midst of my praying I began to sing. I first sang the lines of a song I knew and then began singing another familiar song right after it. Back and forth between the two songs I went, praising and worshiping God:

> *"Turn your eyes upon Jesus*
> *Look full in His wonderful face*
> *And the things of earth will grow strangely dim*
> *In the light of His glory and grace."*
> *"Jesus, Jesus, Jesus*
> *There's just something about that name*
> *Master, Savior, Jesus*
> *Like the fragrance after the rain*
> *Jesus, Jesus, Jesus*
> *Let all Heaven and earth proclaim*

Kings and kingdoms shall all pass away
But there's something about that name."

Back and forth between the songs I went. I was in a state of adoration to our Lord, when all of a sudden, in the middle of the first song, I began singing in a language that began to flow from me in a melody unlike anything I had ever heard! And it was so natural! The more I worshipped, the more that melody soared and poured out from me. I was in awe, and yet it was totally natural! As I sang this heavenly song, the Lord began putting the words in English right in front of me. They scrolled in front of me like the shape of a rainbow. I was singing in an unknown language, yet I was seeing it scrolled out in front of me in English! It was all so incredible, yet all so natural. It seemed like a normal part of who I was and as if I had been doing it all my life!

This went on for about fifteen minutes before I stopped. I sat there and said to myself, Did I just sing in tongues? Is singing in tongues even possible? Then I began to pray and thank God for what had just occurred when all of a sudden my prayer went from English into a language I had never heard before! The more I prayed, the more it poured out of me like a river! I couldn't stop!

I didn't want to stop! Finally, after about ten more minutes of speaking in this unknown language, I stopped. I was so overwhelmed and yet excited at the same time. I was also very anxious to tell Linda, so I went back into the house; but she was sound asleep. I crawled into bed and just lay there in wonderment about what had just occurred. I thought to myself, Have I been baptized in the Holy Spirit? Can I speak in this unknown language again if I want? So lying there in my bed, I began to quietly pray again. And sure enough, it poured out of me! I was so excited, yet so at peace. I fell asleep with a sense of awe and wonder at what a great God we serve!

The next morning I told Linda what had happened. She was so excited for me and yet disappointed that she had not yet experienced the Baptism of the Spirit for herself. Her time was yet to come! That evening I got on the phone and called Pastor Buddy. When he answered, I told him I had something to tell him. Immediately he got all choked up and started crying! I asked him what he was crying about, and he said that he knew what I was going to tell him already! I asked him, "What!?" And he told me that he knew that I had received the gift of the Spirit! Then I proceeded to tell him the whole story. We cried and rejoiced together on the phone that evening.

Friends, I had been operating on only four cylinders for all the years I was in ministry! Take it from a man who had been raised to believe that the Baptism of the Holy Spirit was not a valid experience. What a trick of the enemy to blind the eyes of believers so that they don't operate with all the power and strength made available to them by God! Let me share some scriptures with you:

> *Acts 1:4-5 (NIV): "⁴On one occasion, while he was eating with them, he gave them this command: 'Do not leave Jerusalem, but wait for the gift my Father promised, which you have heard me speak about. ⁵For John baptized with water, but in a few days you will be baptized with the Holy Spirit."*
>
> *Acts 11:15-17 (NIV): " ¹⁵As I began to speak, the Holy Spirit came on them as he had come on us at the beginning. ¹⁶Then I remembered what the Lord had said: 'John baptized with water, but you will be baptized with the Holy Spirit.'*
>
> *¹⁷So if God gave them the same gift as he gave us, who believed in the Lord Jesus Christ, who was I to think that I could oppose God?"*
>
> *Acts 2:4 (NIV): "⁴All of them were filled with the Holy Spirit and began to speak in other tongues as the Spirit enabled them."*
>
> *Acts 19:6 (NIV): "⁶When Paul placed his hands on them, the Holy Spirit came on them, and they spoke in tongues and prophesied."*

1 Corinthians 12:5-11 (NIV): "⁵There are differ-ent kinds of service, but the same Lord.

⁶There are different kinds of working, but the same God works all of them in all men.

⁷Now to each one the manifestation of the Spirit is given for the common good.

⁸To one there is given through the Spirit the mes-sage of wisdom, to another the message of knowl-edge by means of the same Spirit,

⁹to another faith by the same Spirit, to another gifts of healing by that one Spirit,

¹⁰to another miraculous powers, to another proph-ecy, to another distinguishing between spirits, to an-other speaking in different kinds of tongues, and to still another the interpretation of tongues.

¹¹All these are the work of one and the same Spir-it, and he gives them to each one, just as he deter-mines."

Not only did I receive the Baptism of the Holy Spirit, but two weeks later at a Sunday night service, my little, "former-Baptist" wife did also! Wow! Talk about a paradigm shift! My prayer life has been transformed; my approach to minis-try has been changed; my heart has been healed; and I have been set free to worship and praise the Lord as never before! I have strength from God that I've never had before or ever thought possible!

Thank you, God, for sending your Son; thank you, Je-sus, for sending your Spirit; thank you, Spirit, for the gift of tongues and any of the other gifts that come from You, which allow us to be used for the Kingdom of God and for His glory!

So, why did God allow me to go through depression? My third answer is that I believe God not only wanted to get me to a place where I was desperate for Him more than any-thing, wanted me to be set free of junk I had carried all my life, and wanted me to be filled with His Holy Spirit and operating in the gifts of the Spirit. He also wanted to move me out of the ministry at the church I had started and pastored for thirteen years.

I had come to believe that long term ministry in one church was the way to go. All the research pointed in that direction. But now I see that part of the ache I carried all those years was not only to be Baptized with His Holy Spirit, but also to see that the church I served all those years was a training ground for Linda and me. It was a place of training, not only for ourselves, but also for those I had raised up to follow and eventually carry on the work.

God wanted us to be able to launch out into even deeper water with our ministry. It was valid and essential to be there during that time, but now God has put an excitement within me that I can hardly contain! It is an excitement to go out and snatch more souls from the enemy's grasp! I have a pastor's heart and love to teach the Word, but I also have an evangelist's fire burning deep within me that wants to be unleashed, that wants to win souls. There is nothing like being part of the process of seeing someone born again into the Kingdom of God! I have been a part of leading many people to Christ in the past, but that is not enough—there are countless more I long to help bring into the fold!

Can I dare tell you what wells up within me twenty-four hours a day, seven days a week, and wants to be unleashed and set free? You may think I am nuts, but I must find out! I cannot be content as long as this fire rages within me!

Because of His great love, which sent my Savior to the cross, it would be a privilege to serve my Lord in the following ways: to preach the Gospel all over the world and watch countless numbers respond to God's call and be saved; to lay hands on the sick and see them healed; to lay hands on the saints of God and watch them receive the Baptism of the Holy Spirit and fire; to impart spiritual gifts through the laying on of hands in order for others to go out and do great things for God; to ordain more and more men and women into the ministry as evangelists for the winning of souls;

to prophesy in the name of the Lord; to raise up an army of believers, who go out in the strength and power of Almighty God and storm the gates of hell for lost souls; to start churches full of consecrated believers, who are set free from sin and are operating in their gifts for the Body of Christ; to perform signs, wonders, and miracles in Jesus' name and for His glory; and to see His FAME spread throughout the earth!

It's a big desire, wouldn't you agree? But why not? Why not me? . . . . . Why not you? What is holding you back from letting go and letting God use you in any way He sees fit? The journey we live for Him is far more exciting than anything we could ever plan and live for ourselves! I've already been through a wonderful adventure these first fifty-four years of my life. But the best is yet to come! I'm certain of it! The old Dave is dead; God has raised up from the ashes of depression a new man in Christ Jesus—one who walks in the power and strength of the Holy Spirit, one whose void has been filled to overflowing.

My former congregation is in the hands of a new group of believers, many of whom I had the privilege to train, raise up, and ordain. How they respond to this moment, to this challenge, is now up to them. They wanted the opportunity—now they've got it. I only pray that in each and every person or congregation I have the privilege of serving, that God will raise them up to be warriors for the Kingdom of God and that they too will storm the gates of hell for the glory of our risen King!

Chapter 33

Why did I write this book? I believe that by reading about the experience I went through, others can be encouraged and find hope in God. It's that simple. So many people are right now battling depression. Maybe you are one of them. You feel as if there is no hope. I know. I've been there. But that is a lie from the enemy, who has come to kill, steal, and destroy the wonderful things God has planned for your life! Maybe you have no support from family, friends, or even the church you attend. You have support from Heaven itself! You may feel abandoned and lost. God knows where you are and doesn't want you to go through this trial alone. He wants to carry you. There was a time I didn't believe this, but I know it now as much as I know anything. He has promised to never leave you nor forsake you!

> *Hebrews 13:5 (NIV): "God has said, 'Never will I leave you; never will I forsake you.'"*
> *Joshua 1:5 (NIV): "No one will be able to stand up against you all the days of your life. As I was with Moses, so I will be with you; I will never leave you nor forsake you."*

Though you feel like no one understands you, God does! Don't give up! If God can bring me through, then He can do it for you!

I believe that a big part of my ministry from here on will be to testify to what God can do in a situation that seems hopeless. When others abandon you and give up on you, God wants to turn the situation around and give you hope and a future. He did it for me, but you have to run to Him with total abandonment and want Jesus more than anything—and I do mean anything!

> *Psalm 34:18 (NIV): "The LORD is close to the bro-kenhearted and saves those who are crushed in spir-*

it." He is near to you, but you have to reach out to Him and seek His face in the hopelessness of your situation. He will hear you!

Psalm 18:5-6 (NIV): "⁵ The cords of the grave coiled around me; the snares of death confronted me.

⁶ In my distress I called to the LORD; I cried to my God for help. From his temple he heard my voice; my cry came before him, into his ears."

So where do I go from here? What is it that God has for Linda and me next? We don't know for sure everything He has planned, but we do know we have been called to minister the Gospel in these "Last Days" before He returns. I also know that we now go out in the strength and power of the Spirit of the Living God. I know we are more equipped to minister than ever before—we have God's anointing, God's call, and two great church families—my current church, "Fountain of Life Church," in Okeechobee, Florida, and Central Assembly in Vero Beach, Florida, with Pastor Buddy Tipton, to support us in our endeavors. We are truly blessed!

I know I have a pastor's heart, but also realize I have a passion for lost souls and a zeal to see countless people come to Christ. I know that I have the call of an evangelist on my life, as well as a fire burning deep within my belly, which cannot be quenched by mere everyday activity, a fire in the deepest recesses of my soul, which rises from a call God placed on my life when I was fifteen years old and is fueled by the presence and power of the Holy Spirit! Where will all this go? Where will we be used next? Isn't it awesome to anticipate the next move of God!? Locally or around the world, we are ready and willing to be used by our wonderful Lord.

Whatever is next is in God's hands, but I know that I must be about my Father's business . . . . . .

Isaiah 61:1 (NIV):
"The Spirit of the Sovereign LORD is on me, because the LORD has anointed me

to preach good news to the poor.
He has sent me to bind up the brokenhearted,
to proclaim freedom for the captives
and release from darkness for the prisoners . . . ."

This is my story . . . . what is yours? Each of us has a story. Lay down any excuses and commit yourself anew to follow Jesus anywhere He leads.

It will be the greatest adventure you will ever take!

Author's Biography

David Robertson and his wife, Linda, live in Okeechobee, Florida. They have three boys and five grandchildren between them. David received his Bachelor's degree in Religion with a double major in Ministry and Missions from Kentucky Mountain Bible College in Vancleve, Kentucky. He then went on to receive another Bachelor's in Education from Morehead State University in Morehead, Kentucky.

David has taught middle school and high school social studies classes for thirty plus years and has been involved in church work of every kind since 1978. He established and was Senior Minister of a church in Okeechobee for thirteen years before resigning in November of 2008 due to his illness. He has since started a new ministry and eventually merged it with an existing church. He is the Senior Minister of Fountain of Life Church in Okeechobee, Florida.

Linda Robertson has worked for the Okeechobee school system for over twenty years and is presently teaching third grade. Linda received her Bachelor's Degree in Elementary Education from Florida Atlantic University. She has been actively involved in church work since 1980, leading women's ministries and directing children's programs.

David and Linda are available for speaking engagements, either to speak about his struggle with depression and ultimate healing or as an evangelist to spread the Good News of God's love.

You may also contact him for speaking engagements through the following means:

e-mail: davidrobertson57@hotmail.com
phone: 863-801-1297
street address:
2153 S.W. 1st Way
Okeechobee, Florida 34974

CPSIA information can be obtained at www.ICGtesting.com
Printed in the USA
LVOW06s1446020913

350624LV00001B/22/P